Sexual Health

Series Editor: Cara Acred

Volume 309

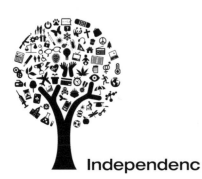

Independenc  blishers

First published by Independence Educational Publishers

The Studio, High Green

Great Shelford

Cambridge CB22 5EG

England

© Independence 2017

Copyright

Photocopy licence

ISBN-13: 978 1 86168 759 3

Printed in Great Britain

Zenith Print Group

Contents

Introduction

Sexual Health is Volume 309 in the **ISSUES** series. The aim of the series is to offer current, diverse information about important issues in our world, from a UK perspective.

ABOUT TITLE

Sexual health is an issue that will always need to be discussed. This book explores traditional topics such as contraception, sexually transmitted diseases and teenage pregnancy. It also looks at sex education in the UK – considering whether our schools are performing well enough in this vital area – and raises questions about topical issues like abstinence pledges, the cervical cancer vaccine and the importance of consent.

OUR SOURCES

Titles in the **ISSUES** series are designed to function as educational resource books, providing a balanced overview of a specific subject.

The information in our books is comprised of facts, articles and opinions from many different sources, including:

⇨ Newspaper reports and opinion pieces

⇨ Website factsheets

⇨ Magazine and journal articles

⇨ Statistics and surveys

⇨ Government reports

⇨ Literature from special interest groups.

A NOTE ON CRITICAL EVALUATION

Because the information reprinted here is from a number of different sources, readers should bear in mind the origin of the text and whether the source is likely to have a particular bias when presenting information (or when conducting their research). It is hoped that, as you read about the many aspects of the issues explored in this book, you will critically evaluate the information presented.

It is important that you decide whether you are being presented with facts or opinions. Does the writer give a biased or unbiased report? If an opinion is being expressed, do you agree with the writer? Is there potential bias to the 'facts' or statistics behind an article?

ASSIGNMENTS

In the back of this book, you will find a selection of assignments designed to help you engage with the articles you have been reading and to explore your own opinions. Some tasks will take longer than others and there is a mixture of design, writing and research-based activities that you can complete alone or in a group.

Useful weblinks

www.aidsmap.com

www.bma.org.uk

www.brook.org.uk

www.centreforsocialjustice.org.uk

www.theconversation.com

www.familylives.org.uk

www.theguardian.com

www.helpage.org

www.huffingtonpost.co.uk

www.ibtimes.co.uk

www.letstalkaboutit.nhs.uk

www.medinstitute.org

www.natcen.ac.uk

www.natsal.ac.uk

www.nhs.uk

www.nspcc.org.uk

www.oxfordonlinepharmacy.co.uk

www.sec-ed.co.uk

www.sexeducationforum.org.uk

www.solent.nhs.uk

www.telegraph.co.uk

www.umbrellahealth.co.uk

www.who.int

www.yougov.co.uk

FURTHER RESEARCH

At the end of each article we have listed its source and a website that you can visit if you would like to conduct your own research. Please remember to critically evaluate any sources that you consult and consider whether the information you are viewing is accurate and unbiased.

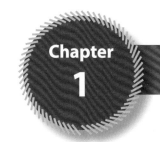

What is sexual health?

Sexual health is a state of physical, mental and social well-being in relation to sexuality. It requires a positive and respectful approach to sexuality and sexual relationships, as well as the possibility of having pleasurable and safe sexual experiences, free of coercion, discrimination and violence.

Defining sexual health

The World Health Organization (WHO) has been working in the area of sexual health since at least 1974, when the deliberations of an expert committee resulted in the publication of a technical report entitled *Education and treatment in human sexuality* (WHO, 1975).

In 2000, the Pan American Health Organization (PAHO) and WHO convened a number of expert consultations to review terminology and identify programme options. In the course of these meetings, the working definitions of key terms used here were developed. In a subsequent meeting, organized by PAHO and the World Association for Sexual Health (WAS), a number of sexual health concerns were addressed with respect to body integrity, sexual safety, eroticism, gender, sexual orientation, emotional attachment and reproduction.

Working definitions

Sex

Sex refers to the biological characteristics that define humans as female or male. While these sets of biological characteristics are not mutually exclusive, as there are individuals who possess both, they tend to differentiate humans as males and females. In general use in many languages, the term sex is often used to mean 'sexual activity', but for technical purposes in the context of sexuality and sexual health discussions, the above definition is preferred.

Sexual health

According to the current working definition, sexual health is:

"…a state of physical, emotional, mental and social well-being in relation to sexuality; it is not merely the absence of disease, dysfunction or infirmity. Sexual health requires a positive and respectful approach to sexuality and sexual relationships, as well as the possibility of having pleasurable and safe sexual experiences, free of coercion, discrimination and violence. For sexual health to be attained and maintained, the sexual rights of all persons must be respected, protected and fulfilled." (WHO, 2006a)

Sexuality

Sexual health cannot be defined, understood or made operational without a broad consideration of sexuality, which underlies important behaviours and outcomes related to sexual health. The working definition of sexuality is:

"…a central aspect of being human throughout life encompasses sex, gender identities and roles, sexual orientation, eroticism, pleasure, intimacy and reproduction. Sexuality is experienced and expressed in thoughts, fantasies, desires, beliefs, attitudes, values, behaviours, practices, roles and relationships. While sexuality can include all of these dimensions, not all of them are always experienced or expressed. Sexuality is influenced by the interaction of biological, psychological, social, economic, political, cultural, legal, historical, religious and spiritual factors." (WHO, 2006a)

Sexual rights

There is a growing consensus that sexual health cannot be achieved and maintained without respect for, and protection of, certain human rights. The working definition of sexual rights given below is a contribution to the continuing dialogue on human rights related to sexual health (1).

"The fulfilment of sexual health is tied to the extent to which human rights are respected, protected and fulfilled. Sexual rights embrace certain human rights that are already recognised in

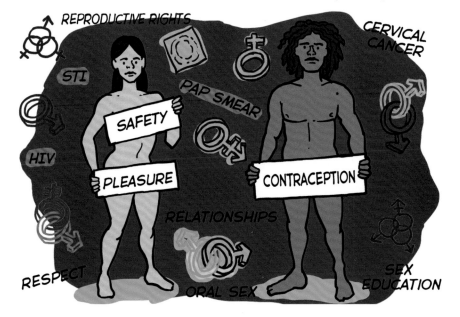

international and regional human rights documents and other consensus documents and in national laws.

Rights critical to the realisation of sexual health include:

⇨ the rights to equality and non-discrimination

⇨ the right to be free from torture or to cruel, inhumane or degrading treatment or punishment

⇨ the right to privacy

⇨ the rights to the highest attainable standard of health (including sexual health) and social security

⇨ the right to marry and to found a family and enter into marriage with the free and full consent of the intending spouses, and to equality in and at the dissolution of marriage

⇨ the right to decide the number and spacing of one's children

⇨ the rights to information, as well as education

⇨ the rights to freedom of opinion and expression, and

⇨ the right to an effective remedy for violations of fundamental rights.

The responsible exercise of human rights requires that all persons respect the rights of others.

The application of existing human rights to sexuality and sexual health constitute sexual rights. Sexual rights protect all people's rights to fulfil and express their sexuality and enjoy sexual health, with due regard for the rights of others and within a framework of protection against discrimination." (WHO, 2006a, updated 2010)

(1) It should be noted that this definition does not represent an official WHO position and should not be used or quoted as such. It is offered instead as a contribution to ongoing discussion about sexual health.

⇨ The above information is reprinted with kind permission from the World Health Organization. Please visit www.who.int for further information.

Sexual health mythbusters

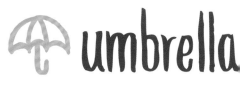

Myth: condoms fail, so I will not use them

Fact: condoms are the most effective way to prevent most sexually transmitted infection (STIs). The most common reason for failure of a condom is not using it correctly.

Myth: I can't use condoms because I'm allergic to latex

Fact: latex-free condoms are available for those who are allergic to latex. Not using condoms greatly increases the risk of catching a sexually transmitted infection (STI).

Myth: I will have to pay for my HIV tests and treatments in the clinics

Fact: all tests and treatments provided in Umbrella clinics are free.

Myth: if I don't have any symptoms, I am clear of STIs

Fact: not everybody with a sexually transmitted infection (STI) shows signs or symptoms of the infection. If left untreated, STIs may result in serious and difficult-to-treat complications.

Myth: if you are a good judge of character you can tell who is infected with STIs

Sexually transmitted infections (STIs) can affect anyone who has had unprotected sex. No one can use their instinct to decide their risk of an STI. Getting tested and regular condom use are the best ways to protect yourself from STIs.

Myth: men who go to sexual health clinics have to have an 'umbrella test' for STIs

We can use urine samples to test for chlamydia and gonorrhoea. If we have to use swabs, they are as small as possible so that apart from momentary nippiness, there will be very little discomfort. You may also be able to take a free STI test at home, using one of our self-sampling kits. STI self-sampling kits

Myth: my partner has had a negative test for everything. I don't need to worry about STIs

Fact: just because your partner is negative you can not assume you are too. Remember, sexually transmitted infections (STIs) may not cause any symptoms. You could have an STI from your previous partner(s) without knowing. The only way you can reliably claim you are negative is to be tested yourself. STI tests do not test for all infections. The 'standard' test if you do not have any symptoms is for chlamydia, gonorrhoea, HIV and syphilis.

Myth: once you've had an STI, there's no chance of getting it again

Fact: you can get some STIs more than just once. For example, infection with chlamydia, gonorrhoea, syphilis or trichomonas vaginalis does not protect you from catching them again.

Myth: oral contraceptive pills protect against STIs

Fact: oral contraceptive pills protect women against becoming pregnant. They can't protect against STIs. Regular use of condoms is the best way to protect against STIs. To be safe against both pregnancy and STIs, it's best to use condoms and for a woman to use another method of contraception – such as the pill – at the same time.

Myth: there is no need to worry about STIs. It only takes a course of antibiotics to get clear

Fact: recent advances have made treatment of many sexually transmitted infections (STIs) easy and very effective. However, every year, due to late diagnosis, a number of infected patients develop STI complications that are difficult to treat. For example, treatment of early chlamydia is simple but untreated infection can lead to pelvic inflammatory disease and infertility, which are very difficult to treat. Also, viral infections, like genital warts and herpes, are more difficult to treat in some people and can keep coming back. It's best to help avoid STIs altogether by using a condom when you have sex.

Myth: we don't need to use condoms because I'm too old to get pregnant

Fact: if you're having sex, you're still at risk of sexually transmitted infections. The best way to prevent the spread of STIs is by using a condom every time you have sex. If you want to be sure you don't already have an STI, get tested.

Myth: only drug users and gay men can catch HIV

Fact: in recent years, more heterosexual men and women have been diagnosed with HIV than gay men and drug users put together. Anyone with a history of unprotected sex may be at risk of HIV, and should therefore be tested.

Myth: you can't catch HIV through oral sex

Fact: wrong. HIV can be spread through oral sex. It's best to use condoms or dental dams for oral sex to reduce the risk of catching HIV.

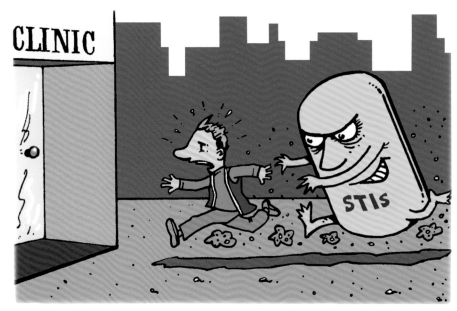

Myth: a woman can't become pregnant if she has sex during her period

Fact: it is true that a woman having her period is not ovulating (releasing egg cells). However, the time of ovulation in women can be irregular. Because sperm can live inside a women's body for five days, a woman who ovulates within seven days after having sex can get pregnant. Having unprotected sex during your period is not a reliable method of contraception.

Myth: a woman will not become pregnant if she takes a shower or bath right after sex, or if she urinates right after sex

Fact: it's possible for a woman to become pregnant if she washes or urinates straight after having sex. Washing or urinating after sex will not stop sperm that have already entered through the cervix (the neck of the womb).

Myth: women on the pill put on weight

Fact: research has not shown any relationship between weight gain and use of the contraceptive pill. The oestrogen in the pill may make some women feel bloated, and the hormone progesterone may increase appetite. Some women seem to put on weight that may be related to their increased appetite, or natural changes in body weight that occur in certain phases of life.

Myth: you can't get pregnant the first time you have sex

Fact: women can get pregnant the first time they have sex. If you are thinking of having sex, you should use a reliable method of contraception and a condom.

Myth: you can use plastic wrap or cling film instead of a condom

Fact: plastic wrap and cling film cannot be used instead of a condom. Condoms are specifically made to provide a good fit and good protection during sex, and they are thoroughly tested for maximum effectiveness.

Myth: you should not take the contraceptive pill for long

Fact: it is believed that the pill can be taken for more than 15 years without risk. Taking a break from the pill may result in you becoming pregnant. If you choose to change from the pill, you should discuss an alternative method of contraception with your doctor.

⇨ The above information is reprinted with kind permission from Umbrella. Please visit www.umbrellahealth. co.uk for further information.

Sexual attitudes and lifestyles in Britain

Highlights from the Nastal report.

We interviewed 15,162 men and women aged 16–74 between September 2010 and August 2012. They provided us with valuable information about their experiences, behaviours and views which will shape our understanding of sexual health in Britain. Here we present highlights from our initial findings. The full articles can be found in *The Lancet* (www.thelancet.com/themed/natsal) and details of the study methodology are on the Natsal website (www.natsal.ac.uk).

Changes in sexual behaviour

This is the third Natsal survey that has been carried out in Britain: the first survey was undertaken in 1990–1991 and the second survey in 1999–2001. Over the 1990s, we saw an increase in the number of opposite-sex partners people reported, and more people reporting same-sex experience. Over the last decade, we have only seen further increases for women, so the gender gap is narrowing.

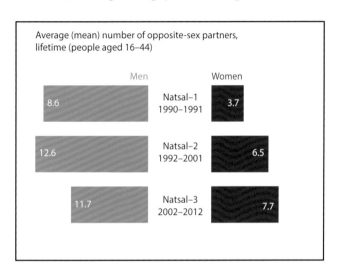

Average (mean) number of opposite-sex partners, lifetime (people aged 16–44)

	Men	Women
Natsal–1 1990–1991	8.6	3.7
Natsal–2 1992–2001	12.6	6.5
Natsal–3 2002–2012	11.7	7.7

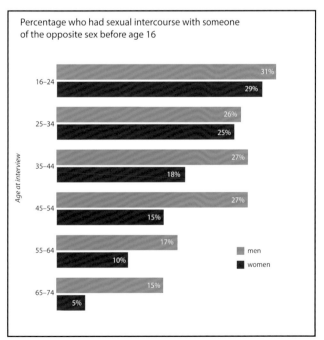

Percentage who had sexual intercourse with someone of the opposite sex before age 16

Age at interview

Age	men	women
16–24	31%	29%
25–34	26%	25%
35–44	27%	18%
45–54	27%	15%
55–64	17%	10%
65–74	15%	5%

Sex and health

Overall, more than 60% of people reported having sex recently and over 60% of people said they were satisfied with their sex life. People in poorer health were less likely to have had sex recently, and less likely to say that they were satisfied. This was true even after taking age and whether people were in a relationship into account. However, ill health does not necessarily mean the end of an active or satisfying sex life: more than one in three people in bad or very bad health had had sex recently, and around half were satisfied with their sex lives.

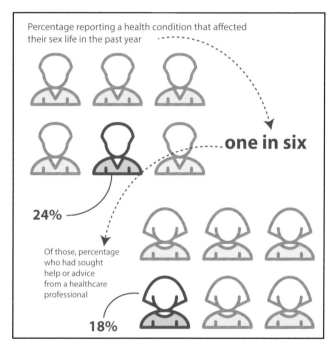

Percentage reporting a health condition that affected their sex life in the past year

one in six

24%

Of those, percentage who had sought help or advice from a healthcare professional

18%

Almost one in six people said they had a health condition that affected their sex life in the past year, yet less than one in four of these men and one in five of these women said that they had tried to get help or advice from a healthcare professional. Those who had were most likely to have talked to their GP.

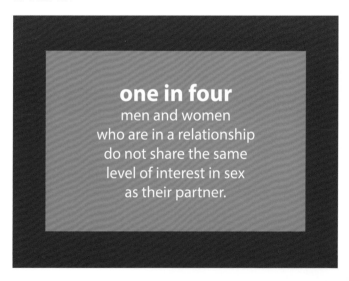

one in four
men and women
who are in a relationship
do not share the same
level of interest in sex
as their partner.

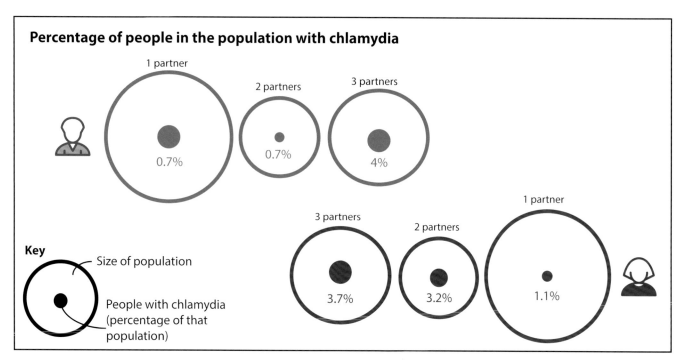

Percentage of people in the population with chlamydia

1 partner — 0.7%

2 partners — 0.7%

3 partners — 4%

3 partners — 3.7%

2 partners — 3.2%

1 partner — 1.1%

Key

Size of population

People with chlamydia (percentage of that population)

Sexually transmitted infections (STIs)

We collected urine from a sample of men and women aged 16–44 which we tested anonymously for sexually transmitted infections (STIs), including chlamydia, gonorrhoea, human papillomavirus (HPV) and HIV. These findings are for men and women who have ever had sex. HPV was the most common STI, followed by chlamydia. HIV and gonorrhoea were found in around one in 1,000 people. For more information about these STIs and where you can test for them you can visit the NHS website: www.nhs.uk/Livewell/STIs/Pages/STIs-hub.aspx.

Overall, around one in 100 people aged 16–44 had chlamydia, although this varied by age, peaking at almost one in 20 women aged 18–19 and one in thirty men aged 20–24. Although people who reported more partners in the past year were more likely to have chlamydia, a lot of the chlamydia was found in people who reported only one partner in the past year, because most people only had one partner.

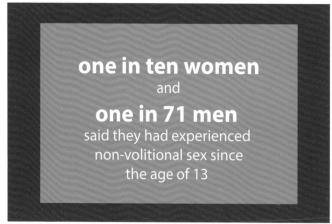

one in ten women
and
one in 71 men
said they had experienced non-volitional sex since the age of 13

Over the past decade, national sexual health strategies in Britain have aimed to increase access to sexual health services and STI / HIV testing. Compared with the previous survey (1999–2001), more people reported having an HIV test or going to a sexual health clinic in the past five years. It is encouraging to see that these increases were even larger in those at highest risk, such as people who reported more partners.

Non-volitional sex

We asked men and women "since the age of 13, has anyone made you have sex with them, against your will?" which we refer to as 'non-volitional sex'. One in ten women and one in 71 men said that they had experienced non-volitional sex since age 13.

⇨ The above information is reprinted with kind permission from Natsal. Please visit www.natsal.ac.uk for further information.

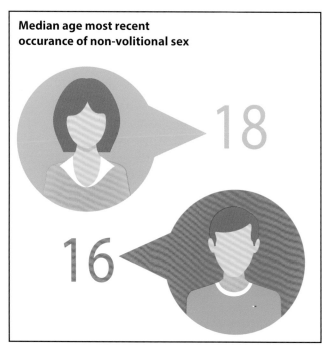

Median age most recent occurance of non-volitional sex

18

16

What is contraception?

Contraception aims to prevent pregnancy. A woman can get pregnant if a man's sperm reaches one of her eggs (ova).

Contraception tries to stop this happening by keeping the egg and sperm apart, or by stopping egg production, or by stopping the combined sperm and egg (fertilised egg) attaching to the lining of the womb.

Contraception is free for most people in the UK. With 15 methods to choose from, you can find one that suits you best.

Barrier methods such as condoms are a form of contraception that help to protect against sexually transmitted infections (STIs) and pregnancy. You should use condoms to protect both your sexual health and that of your partner, no matter what the other contraception you're using to prevent pregnancy.

The 15 methods of contraception

Don't be put off if the first type you use isn't quite right – you can try another. Read about the different methods of contraception:

Caps

The contraceptive cap is a circular dome made of thin, soft silicone (they used to be made of latex, but if you get a cap on the NHS today it will be made of silicone). It's inserted into the vagina before sex, and covers the cervix so that sperm cannot get into the womb. You need to use spermicide with it (spermicide kills sperm).

The cap must be left in place for six hours after sex. After that time, you take out the cap and wash it. Caps are reusable. They come in different sizes, and you must be fitted for the correct size by a trained doctor or nurse.

Combined pill

The combined oral contraceptive pill is usually just called "the pill". It contains artificial versions of the female hormones oestrogen and progesterone, which women produce naturally in their ovaries.

The hormones in the pill prevent your ovaries from releasing an egg (ovulating).

They also make it difficult for sperm to reach an egg, or for an egg to implant itself in the lining of the womb. The pill is usually taken to prevent pregnancy, but can also be used to treat painful periods, heavy periods, premenstrual syndrome (PMS) and endometriosis.

Condoms (female)

Female condoms are made from thin, soft plastic called polyurethane (some male condoms are made from this too). Female condoms are worn inside the vagina to prevent semen getting to the womb.

When used correctly during vaginal sex, they help to protect against pregnancy and sexually transmitted infections (STIs). Condoms are the only contraception that protect against pregnancy and STIs. Currently, there is only one brand of female condom available in the UK, called Femidom.

Condoms (male)

There are two types of condoms: male condoms, which are worn on the penis, and female condoms, which are worn inside the vagina. This section is about male condoms, where you can get them and how they work.

Male condoms are made from very thin latex (rubber), polyisoprene or polyurethane, and are designed to stop a man's semen from coming into contact with his sexual partner.

When condoms are used correctly during vaginal sex, they help to protect against pregnancy and sexually transmitted infections (STIs).

When used correctly during anal and oral sex, they help to protect against STIs. Condoms are the only contraception that protect against pregnancy and STIs.

Contraceptive implant

The contraceptive implant is a small flexible tube about 40mm long that's inserted under the skin of your upper arm. It's inserted by a trained professional, such as a doctor, and lasts for three years.

The implant stops the release of an egg from the ovary by slowly releasing progestogen into your body. Progestogen also thickens the cervical mucus and thins the womb lining. This

makes it harder for sperm to move through your cervix, and less likely for your womb to accept a fertilised egg.

Contraceptive injection

There are three types of contraceptive injections in the UK: Depo-Provera, which lasts for 12 weeks, Sayana Press, which lasts for 13 weeks, and Noristerat, which lasts for eight weeks. The most popular is Depo-Provera. Noristerat is usually used for only short periods of time – for example, if your partner is waiting for a vasectomy.

The injection contains progestogen. This thickens the mucus in the cervix, stopping sperm reaching an egg. It also thins the womb lining and, in some, prevents the release of an egg.

Contraceptive patch

The contraceptive patch is a sticky patch, a bit like a nicotine patch, measuring 5x5cm. It delivers hormones into your body through your skin. In the UK, the patch's brand name is Evra.

It contains the same hormones as the combined pill, and it works in the same way. This means that it prevents ovulation (the release of an egg); it thickens cervical mucus, which makes it more difficult for sperm to travel through the cervix; and it thins the womb lining, making it less likely that a fertilised egg will implant there.

Diaphragms

A contraceptive diaphragm is inserted into the vagina before sex, and it covers the cervix so that sperm can't get into the womb (uterus). You need to use spermicide with it (spermicides kill sperm).

The diaphragm must be left in place for at least six hours after sex. After that time, you take out the diaphragm and wash it (they're reusable). Diaphragms come in different sizes – you must be fitted for the correct size by a trained doctor or nurse.

Intrauterine device (IUD)

An IUD is a small T-shaped plastic and copper device that's inserted into your womb (uterus) by a specially trained doctor or nurse.

The IUD works by stopping the sperm and egg from surviving in the womb or fallopian tubes. It may also prevent a fertilised egg from implanting in the womb.

The IUD is a long-acting reversible contraceptive (LARC) method. This means that once it's in place, you don't have to think about it each day or each time you have sex. There are several types and sizes of IUD.

You can use an IUD whether or not you've had children.

Intrauterine system (IUS)

An IUS is a small, T-shaped plastic device that is inserted into your womb (uterus) by a specially trained doctor or nurse.

The IUS releases a progestogen hormone into the womb. This thickens the mucus from your cervix, making it difficult for sperm to move through and reach an egg. It also thins the womb lining so that it's less likely to accept a fertilised egg. It may also stop ovulation (the release of an egg) in some women.

The IUS is a long-acting reversible contraceptive (LARC) method. It works for five years or three years, depending on the type, so you don't have to think about contraception every day or each time you have sex. Two brands of IUS are used in the UK – Mirena and Jaydess.

You can use an IUS whether or not you've had children.

Natural family planning

Natural family planning is a method that teaches you at what time during the month you can have sex without contraception and with a reduced risk of pregnancy. The method is sometimes called fertility awareness.

It works by plotting the times of the month when you're fertile and when you're not. You learn how to record fertility signals, such as your body temperature and cervical secretions (fluids or mucus), to identify when it's safer to have sex. Natural family planning is more effective when more than one fertility signal is monitored.

You can't learn natural family planning from a book. It has to be learned from a specialist teacher.

Progestogen-only pill

Contains the hormone progestogen, but doesn't contain oestrogen.

You need to take the progestogen-only pill at or around the same time every day.

The progestogen-only pill thickens the mucus in the cervix, which stops sperm reaching an egg. In can also stop ovulation, depending on the type of progestogen-only pill you take.

Newer progestogen-only pills contain desogestrel.

Vaginal ring

The vaginal ring is a small, soft plastic ring that you place inside your vagina. It's about 4mm thick and 5.5cm in diameter. You leave it in your vagina for 21 days, then remove it and throw it in the bin (not down the toilet) in a special disposal bag. Seven days after removing the ring, you insert a new one for the next 21 days.

The ring releases oestrogen and progestogen. This prevents ovulation (release of an egg), makes it difficult for sperm to get to an egg and thins the womb lining, so it's less likely that an egg will implant there.

There are two permanent methods of contraception

Female sterilisation

Female sterilisation is usually carried out under general anaesthetic, but can be carried out under local anaesthetic, depending on the method used. The surgery involves blocking or sealing the fallopian tubes, which link the ovaries to the womb (uterus).

This prevents the woman's eggs from reaching sperm and becoming fertilised. Eggs will still be released from the ovaries as normal, but they will be absorbed naturally into the woman's body.

Male sterilisation (vasectomy)

During a minor operation, the tubes that carry sperm from a man's testicles to the penis are cut, blocked or sealed.

This prevents sperm from reaching the seminal fluid (semen), which is ejaculated from the penis during sex. There will be no sperm in the semen, so a woman's egg can't be fertilised.

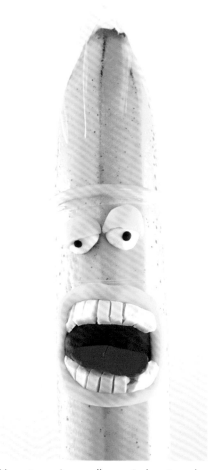

Vasectomy is usually carried out under local anaesthetic, and takes about 15 minutes.

Where to get contraception

Contraceptive services are free and confidential. This includes services for people under 16, as long as they're mature enough to understand the information and decisions involved – there are strict guidelines for healthcare professionals who work with people under 16.

You can get contraception for free from:

⇨ most GP surgeries (talk to your GP or practice nurse)

⇨ community contraception clinics

⇨ some genitourinary medicine (GUM) clinics

⇨ sexual health clinics (these offer contraceptive and STI testing services)

⇨ some young people's services.

Find local sexual health services, including contraception clinics. Or call the national sexual health help line on 0300 123 7123.

Many of these services also offer information, testing and treatment for STIs. If you've had unprotected sex and think there's a chance you might get pregnant, you're also at risk of catching an STI.

Before you make an appointment, try to find out as much as possible about the contraceptive options available. Your choice of contraception may vary over time, depending on your lifestyle and circumstances.

You can find out more about each type of contraception by contacting:

⇨ Brook: the young people's sexual health charity for under-25s

⇨ FPA: provides information on methods of contraception, common STIs, pregnancy choices, abortion, and planning a pregnancy.

What is the male pill?

Ongoing research

There are many ongoing research projects into different methods of male contraception.

Researchers are optimistic that a safe, effective and reversible method of male contraception will eventually become a reality, although this is still several years away.

Types of research

There are two main areas of research into male contraception:

⇨ hormonal contraception – where synthetic (man-made) hormones are used to temporarily stop the development of healthy sperm

⇨ non-hormonal methods – where other techniques are used to prevent healthy sperm from entering a woman's vagina.

Hormonal contraception

In fertile men, new sperm cells are constantly created in the testicles. This process is triggered by the hormone testosterone.

The goal of hormonal contraception research is to find a way of temporarily blocking the effects of testosterone so testicles stop producing healthy sperm cells. However, this needs to be achieved without lowering testosterone levels to such an extent that it triggers side effects,

such as a loss of sexual desire.

Synthetic testosterone and other steroid combinations

One way of doing this is by giving men a synthetic version of testosterone, together with a hormone called progestogen. Progestogens are synthetic versions of a female sex hormone often found in female hormonal contraceptives, such as the progestogen-only pill.

This approach stops the testes producing testosterone which, in most cases, prevents normal sperm production. However, at the same time it keeps the amount of testosterone in the blood normal, preventing side effects.

This is a very effective approach, but some men still carry on producing enough sperm to cause a pregnancy. The reason why this happens is unknown, but it may be that some men carry on producing enough testosterone to continue to stimulate some sperm production.

Research is now focusing on different combinations of synthetic testosterone and progestogens. Several trials in different countries are looking at the effectiveness and long-term safety of hormonal contraceptives for men, including some phase III trials. Phase III trials are the last clinical trials carried out before a medicine is given a marketing licence.

An important disadvantage of using synthetic testosterone is that sperm production is suppressed at different rates in men of different ethnic origins.

These differences may be due to genetic, dietary or environmental factors, but the exact reasons are unknown. Understanding the reasons may lead to new ways of providing effective contraception for all men of diverse ethnic backgrounds.

Non-hormonal contraception

Many of the non-hormonal methods of contraception currently being studied involve the vas deferens. The vas deferens is the tube that sperm pass through on their way to the penis. This tube is cut during a vasectomy.

RISUG and the IVD

One promising avenue of research is a technique called reversible inhibition of sperm under guidance (RISUG). During this technique, a non-toxic synthetic chemical is injected into the vas deferens.

The chemical reacts and blocks the vas deferens. It also kills sperm when they come into contact with it. The chemical is effective almost immediately after it is injected.

The chemical stays in place until a man decides that he wants to have children. It can then be washed out using another injection which dissolves and flushes it out of the vas deferens.

A variation of this technique is the intra-vas device (IVD). It involves injecting a "plug" into the vas deferens which can be removed later. The IVD filters out the sperm as it passes through the vas deferens.

Initial results of RISUG and IVD are promising, but further research is needed to assess the long-term effectiveness and safety of both techniques.

Research published in 2013 found that blocking certain proteins in the bodies of male mice rendered them infertile, but did not affect their sexual behaviour or the quality of their sperm. It prevented the sperm cells from being launched during ejaculation. When the mice's sperm was used to artificially inseminate female mice, it resulted in pregnancies and healthy baby mice.

If a way can be found to block these proteins in human males, this may take research a step closer to producing a male contraceptive pill. However, the research is in the very early stages and a male pill has not been developed. You can find out more about the research into proteins, mice and sperm on the NHS Choices website.

Epididymis

Other research is focusing on the epididymis. This is a long, coiled tube behind the testicles that allows sperm to mature normally, which is essential for normal fertility.

Attempts have been made to interfere with the way the epididymis works and the way sperm matures inside the epididymis. However, so far neither approach has been successful.

⇨ The above information is reprinted with kind permission from NHS Choices. Please visit www.nhs.uk for further information.

Sexually transmitted infections (STIs)

Key facts

⇨ More than one million sexually transmitted infections (STIs) are acquired every day worldwide.

⇨ Each year, there are an estimated 357 million new infections with one of four STIs: chlamydia, gonorrhoea, syphilis and trichomoniasis.

⇨ More than 500 million people are estimated to have genital infection with herpes simplex virus (HSV).

⇨ More than 290 million women have a human papillomavirus (HPV) infection[1].

⇨ The majority of STIs have no symptoms or only mild symptoms that may not be recognised as an STI.

⇨ STIs such as HSV type 2 and syphilis can increase the risk of HIV acquisition.

⇨ Over 900,000 pregnant women were infected with syphilis resulting in approximately 350,000 adverse birth outcomes including stillbirth in 2012[2].

⇨ In some cases, STIs can have serious reproductive health consequences beyond the immediate impact of the infection itself (e.g. infertility or mother-to-child transmission)

⇨ Drug resistance, especially for gonorrhoea, is a major threat to reducing the impact of STIs worldwide.

What are sexually transmitted infections and how are they transmitted?

More than 30 different bacteria, viruses and parasites are known to be transmitted through sexual contact. Eight of these pathogens are linked to the greatest incidence of sexually transmitted disease. Of these eight infections, four are currently curable: syphilis, gonorrhoea, chlamydia and trichomoniasis. The other four are viral infections and are incurable: hepatitis B, herpes simplex virus (HSV or herpes), HIV and human papillomavirus (HPV). Symptoms or disease due to the incurable viral infections can be reduced or modified through treatment.

STIs are spread predominantly by sexual contact, including vaginal, anal and oral sex. Some STIs can also be spread through non-sexual means such as via blood or blood products. Many STIs – including chlamydia, gonorrhoea, primarily hepatitis B, HIV, and syphilis – can also be transmitted from mother to child during pregnancy and childbirth.

A person can have an STI without having obvious symptoms of disease. Common symptoms of STIs include vaginal discharge, urethral discharge or burning in men, genital ulcers, and abdominal pain.

Scope of the problem

STIs have a profound impact on sexual and reproductive health worldwide.

More than one million STIs are acquired every day. Each year, there are estimated 357 million new infections with one of four STIs: chlamydia (131 million), gonorrhoea (78 million), syphilis (5.6 million) and trichomoniasis (143 million). More than 500 million people are living with genital HSV (herpes) infection. At any point in time, more than 290 million women have an HPV infection, one of the most common STIs.

STIs can have serious consequences beyond the immediate impact of the infection itself.

⇨ STIs like herpes and syphilis can increase the risk of HIV acquisition three-fold or more.

⇨ Mother-to-child transmission of STIs can result in stillbirth, neonatal death, low birth weight and prematurity, sepsis, pneumonia, neonatal conjunctivitis and congenital deformities. Over 900,000 pregnant women were infected with syphilis resulting in approximately 350,000 adverse birth outcomes including stillbirth in 2012[2].

⇨ HPV infection causes 528,000 cases of cervical cancer and 266,000 cervical cancer deaths each year.

⇨ STIs such as gonorrhoea and chlamydia are major causes of pelvic inflammatory disease (PID) and infertility in women.

Prevention of STIs

Counselling and behavioural approaches

Counselling and behavioural interventions offer primary prevention against STIs (including HIV), as well as against unintended pregnancies. These include:

⇨ comprehensive sexuality education, STI and HIV pre- and post-test counselling;

⇨ safer sex/risk-reduction counselling, condom promotion;

⇨ interventions targeted at key populations, such as sex workers, men who have sex with men and people who inject drugs; and

⇨ education and counselling tailored to the needs of adolescents.

In addition, counselling can improve people's ability to recognise the symptoms of STIs and increase the likelihood they will seek care or encourage a sexual partner to do so. Unfortunately, lack of public awareness, lack of training of health workers, and long-standing, widespread stigma around STIs remain barriers to greater and more effective use of these interventions.

Barrier methods

When used correctly and consistently, condoms offer one of the most effective methods of protection against STIs, including HIV. Female condoms are effective and safe, but are not used as widely by national programmes as male condoms.

Diagnosis of STIs

Accurate diagnostic tests for STIs are widely used in high-income countries. These are especially useful for the diagnosis of asymptomatic infections. However, in low- and middle-income countries, diagnostic tests are largely

1 *Worldwide prevalence and genotype distribution of cervical human papillomavirus DNA in women with normal cytology: a meta-analysis.* de Sanjosé S, Diaz M, Castellsagué X, Clifford G, Bruni L, Muñoz N, et al. Lancet Infect Dis. 2007 Jul;7(7):453-9.

2 *Global Estimates of Syphilis in Pregnancy and Associated Adverse Outcomes: Analysis of Multinational Antenatal Surveillance Data* Newman L, Kamb M, Hawkes S, Gomez G, Say L, Seuc A, et al. PLoS Med 10(2): e1001396. doi:10.1371/journal.pmed.1001396

unavailable. Where testing is available, it is often expensive and geographically inaccessible; and patients often need to wait a long time (or need to return) to receive results. As a result, follow up can be impeded and care or treatment can be incomplete.

The only inexpensive, rapid tests currently available for STIs are for syphilis and HIV. The syphilis test is already in use in some resource-limited settings. The test is accurate, can provide results in 15 to 20 minutes, and is easy to use with minimal training. Rapid syphilis tests have been shown to increase the number of pregnant women tested for syphilis. However, increased efforts are still needed in most low- and middle-income countries to ensure that all pregnant women receive a syphilis test.

Several rapid tests for other STIs are under development and have the potential to improve STI diagnosis and treatment, especially in resource-limited settings.

Treatment of STIs

Effective treatment is currently available for several STIs.

⇨ Three bacterial STIs (chlamydia, gonorrhoea and syphilis) and one parasitic STI (trichomoniasis) are generally curable with existing, effective single-dose regimens of antibiotics.

⇨ For herpes and HIV, the most effective medications available are antivirals that can modulate the course of the disease, though they cannot cure the disease.

⇨ For hepatitis B, immune system modulators (interferon) and antiviral medications can help to fight the virus and slow damage to the liver.

Resistance of STIs – in particular gonorrhoea – to antibiotics has increased rapidly in recent years and has reduced treatment options. The emergence of decreased susceptibility of gonorrhoea to the 'last line' treatment option (oral and injectable cephalosporins) together with antimicrobial resistance already shown to penicillins, sulphonamides, tetracyclines, quinolones and macrolides make gonorrhoea a multidrug-resistant organism. Antimicrobial resistance for other STIs, though less common, also exists, making prevention and prompt treatment critical.

STI case management

Low- and middle-income countries rely on identifying consistent, easily recognizable signs and symptoms to guide treatment, without the use of laboratory tests. This is called syndromic management. This approach, which often relies on clinical algorithms, allows health workers to diagnose a specific infection on the basis of observed syndromes (e.g. vaginal discharge, urethral discharge, genital ulcers, abdominal pain).

Syndromic management is simple, assures rapid, same-day treatment, and avoids expensive or unavailable diagnostic tests. However, this approach misses infections that do not demonstrate any syndromes - the majority of STIs globally.

Vaccines and other biomedical interventions

Safe and highly effective vaccines are available for two STIs: hepatitis B and HPV. These vaccines have represented major advances in STI prevention. The vaccine against hepatitis B is included in infant immunisation programmes in 93% of countries and has already prevented an estimated 1.3 million deaths from chronic liver disease and cancer.

HPV vaccine is available as part of routine immunisation programmes in 65 countries, most of them high- and middle-income. HPV vaccination could prevent the deaths of more than four million women over the next decade in low- and middle-income countries, where most cases of cervical cancer occur, if 70% vaccination coverage can be achieved.

Research to develop vaccines against herpes and HIV is advanced, with several vaccine candidates in early clinical development. Research into vaccines for chlamydia, gonorrhoea, syphilis and trichomoniasis is in earlier stages of development.

Other biomedical interventions to prevent some STIs include adult male circumcision and microbicides.

⇨ Male circumcision reduces the risk of heterosexually acquired HIV infection in men by approximately 60% and provides some protection against other STIs, such as herpes and HPV.

⇨ Tenofovir gel, when used as a vaginal microbicide, has had mixed results in terms of the ability to prevent HIV acquisition, but has shown some effectiveness against HSV-2.

Current efforts to contain the spread of STIs are not sufficient

Behaviour change is complex

Despite considerable efforts to identify simple interventions that can reduce risky sexual behaviour, behaviour change remains a complex challenge. Research has demonstrated the need to focus on carefully defined populations, consult extensively with the identified target populations, and involve them in design, implementation and evaluation.

Health services for screening and treatment of STIs remain weak

People seeking screening and treatment for STIs face numerous problems. These include limited resources, stigmatisation, poor quality of services, and little or no follow-up of sexual partners.

⇨ In many countries, STI services are provided separately and not available in primary healthcare, family planning and other routine health services.

⇨ In many settings, services are often unable to provide screening for asymptomatic infections, lacking trained personnel, laboratory capacity and adequate supplies of appropriate medicines.

⇨ Marginalized populations with the highest rates of STIs – such as sex workers, men who have sex with men, people who inject drugs, prison inmates, mobile populations and adolescents – often do not have access to adequate health services.

August 2016

⇨ The above information is reprinted with kind permission from the World Health Organization. Please visit www.who.int for further information.

Information about common STIs

Chlamydia

Chlamydia is the most common STI in the UK. It is easily passed on during sex. Most people don't experience any symptoms, so they are unaware they're infected.

In women, chlamydia can cause pain or a burning sensation when urinating, a vaginal discharge, pain in the lower abdomen during or after sex, and bleeding during or after sex or between periods.

In men, chlamydia can cause pain or a burning sensation when urinating, a discharge from the tip of the penis, and pain or tenderness in the testicles.

It is also possible to have a chlamydia infection in your rectum (bottom), throat or eyes

Diagnosing chlamydia is done with a urine test or by taking a swab of the affected area. The infection is easily treated with antibiotics but can lead to serious long-term health problems if left untreated, including infertility.

Genital herpes

Genital herpes is a common infection caused by the herpes simplex virus (HSV), which is the same virus that causes cold sores.

Some people develop symptoms of Herpes a few days after coming into contact with the virus. Small, painful blisters or sores usually develop, which may cause itching or tingling, or make it painful to urinate.

After you've been infected, the virus remains dormant (inactive) most of the time. However, certain triggers can reactivate the virus, causing the blisters to develop again, although they're usually smaller and less painful.

It's easier to test for HSV if you have symptoms. Although there's no cure for genital herpes, the symptoms can usually be controlled using antiviral medicines.

If you are diagnosed with herpes, it is important to discuss this with your partner; the staff in the clinic can help support you with this if necessary.

Genital warts

Genital warts are small fleshy growths, bumps or skin changes that appear on or around your genital or anal area. They're caused by the human papilloma virus (HPV) and are the second most common STI in the UK.

Warts are usually painless, but you may notice some itching and discomfort. Occasionally, they can cause bleeding.

You don't need to have penetrative sex to pass the infection on because HPV is spread by skin-to-skin contact.

Several treatments are available for genital warts, including creams and freezing treatment (cryotherapy).

Gonorrhoea

Gonorrhoea is a bacterial STI easily passed on during sex. About 50% of women and 10% of men don't experience any symptoms and are unaware they're infected.

In women, gonorrhoea can cause pain or a burning sensation when urinating, a vaginal discharge (often watery, yellow or green), pain in the lower abdomen during or after sex, and bleeding during or after sex or between periods, sometimes causing heavy periods.

In men, gonorrhoea can cause pain or a burning sensation when urinating, a white, yellow or green discharge from the tip of the penis, and pain or tenderness in the testicles.

It is also possible to have a gonorrhoea infection in your rectum, throat or eyes.

Gonorrhoea is diagnosed using a urine test or by taking a swab of the affected area. The infection is easily treated with antibiotics, but can lead to serious long-term health problems if left untreated, including infertility.

Hepatitis B

Hepatitis B is very infectious (100 times more infectious than HIV) and very easily transmitted through unprotected sex or by sharing needles to inject drugs. Most people who contract hepatitis B do not have symptoms. If symptoms do occur they can appear one to six months after coming into contact with the virus. The infection can persist for many years and silently cause severe liver damage, including cirrhosis, liver failure and liver cancer.

In most people a full course of vaccination prevents infection.

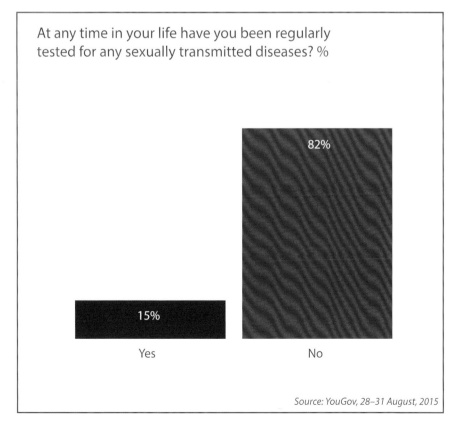

At any time in your life have you been regularly tested for any sexually transmitted diseases? %

82% — No

15% — Yes

Source: YouGov, 28–31 August, 2015

The following people should consider having the hepatitis B vaccination:

⇨ Men who have sex with men

⇨ Anyone who has recently injected drugs

⇨ Anyone who has been paid for sex

⇨ Anyone who has a sexual partner with hepatitis B infection

⇨ Anyone who has been recently sexually assaulted.

HIV

HIV is most commonly passed on through unprotected sex. It can also be transmitted by coming into contact with infected blood – for example, sharing needles to inject drugs or steroids.

The HIV virus attacks and weakens the immune system, making it less able to fight infections and disease. There's no cure for HIV, but there are treatments that allow most people to live a long and otherwise healthy life.

AIDS is the final stage of an HIV infection, when your body can no longer fight life-threatening infections.

Most people with HIV look and feel healthy and have no symptoms. When you first develop HIV, you may experience a flu-like illness with a fever, sore throat or rash. This is called a seroconversion illness.

A simple blood test is usually used to test for an HIV infection. In our clinics we also offer a rapid test using

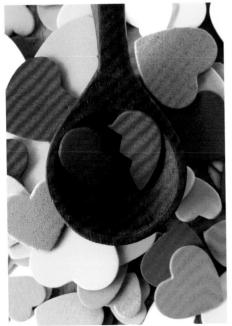

a finger-prick blood test if you are at higher risk of HIV.

Molluscum contagiosum

Molluscum contagiosum is a common and generally harmless viral infection of the skin. It is contagious (can be caught from another person by direct contact). It is most common in children and young adults, but can occur at any age.

Usually the symptoms of these are skin lesions (spots), which are asymptomatic, but the spots can be itchy or sore if they become inflamed or infected. They can bleed slightly if scratched.

Pubic lice

Pubic lice ('crabs') are easily passed to others through close genital contact. They're usually found in pubic hair, but can live in underarm hair, body hair, beards and occasionally eyebrows or eyelashes.

The lice crawl from hair to hair. It may take several weeks for you to notice any symptoms. Most people experience itching and you may notice the lice or eggs on the hairs.

Pubic lice can be successfully treated with special creams or shampoos available over the counter in most pharmacies, from your GP or sexual health clinic. You don't need to shave off your pubic hair or body hair.

Scabies

Scabies is caused by tiny mites that burrow into the skin. It can be passed on through close body or sexual contact, or from infected clothing, bedding or towels.

If you develop scabies, you may have intense itching that's worse at night. The itching can be in your genital area, but it also often occurs between your fingers, on wrists and ankles, under your arms, or on your body and breasts.

You may have a rash or tiny spots. In some people, scabies can be confused with eczema. It's usually very difficult to see the mites.

Scabies can be successfully treated using special creams or shampoos available over the counter in most pharmacies, from a GP or sexual health clinic. The itching can sometimes continue for a short period, even after effective treatment.

Syphilis

Syphilis is a bacterial infection that in the early stages causes a painless, but highly infectious, sore on your genitals. The sore can last up to six weeks before disappearing.

Secondary symptoms such as a rash and a flu-like illness may then develop. These may disappear within a few weeks, after which you'll have no symptoms.

The late (tertiary) stage of syphilis usually occurs after many years, and can cause serious conditions such as heart problems, paralysis and blindness.

The symptoms of syphilis can be difficult to recognise. A simple blood test can be used to diagnose syphilis at any stage. The condition can be treated with antibiotics, usually penicillin injections. When syphilis is treated properly, the later stages can be prevented.

Trichomoniasis

Trichomoniasis is an STI caused by a tiny parasite called *Trichomonas vaginalis* (TV). It can be easily passed on through sex and most people don't know they're infected.

In women, trichomoniasis can cause a frothy yellow or watery vaginal discharge that has an unpleasant smell, soreness or itching around the vagina, and pain when passing urine.

In men, trichomoniasis rarely causes symptoms. You may experience pain or burning after passing urine, a whitish discharge, or an inflamed foreskin.

Trichomoniasis can sometimes be difficult to diagnose but in our clinics we are experienced at diagnosing this infection. We use a microscope to do this. Once diagnosed, it can be treated with antibiotics.

⇨ The above information is reprinted with kind permission from the Solent NHS Trust. Please visit www.letstalkaboutit.nhs.uk or www.solent.nhs.uk for further information.

Which viral STIs are curable and which are incurable?

Herpes and HIV

These are the only two viral STIs which are always chronic. Even though people with herpes or HIV cannot currently be cured, their symptoms can be treated. At this time, there are no available vaccines to prevent Herpes or HIV. However, there are medications available to help prevent the HIV virus from causing infection in the sexual partners of HIV-positive people[1].

HPV

About nine out of ten sexually active people will become infected with the human papillomavirus at some point in their lives. Up to 90% of HPV infections are cleared by the body's immune system within 12–24 months of detection.[2] Some types of HPV are low-risk for cancer, but can cause genital warts. Those who are infected with high-risk (cancer-causing) HPV types and do not clear their infection quickly are at risk for persistent infection. There is no cure for persistent HPV. Persistent HPV infection is a risk factor for development of cervical cancer and oral cancer in men. All women should have routine pap smears by age 21.

There are three available vaccines to help prevent HPV infections. Each of the vaccines needs to be given in a three-part series over a period of six months. The most recent vaccine, Gardasil 9, protects against 9 different strains of the HPV virus, including some of the cancer-causing types and some of the wart-causing types. Both girls and boys are encouraged to be immunized with the vaccines. The vaccine can be given as early as age nine[3].

Hepatitis B

In the U.S., babies usually get their first dose of hepatitis B vaccine at birth and then two more doses of the vaccine by the time they are 18 months old. Adults who were born before 1991 may not have received the vaccine. They should be vaccinated if they are at risk for Hepatitis B exposure[4].

Most adults who are infected with hepatitis B virus (HBV) recover from their infections; the rest develop chronic infections. Each year 2,000-4,000 people in the US die from cirrhosis or liver cancer caused by hepatitis B.[4]

Hepatitis C

There is no vaccine to prevent Hepatitis C. About 75–85% of people infected with Hepatitis C will develop chronic hepatitis C and 60–70% will develop chronic liver disease[5]. Hepatitis C is spread through the blood, but can be sexually transmitted.

Hepatitis C can be cured with medication, especially if the treatment begins within six months of getting the disease. Since 2013, more medications have been approved for use in chronic hepatitis C, resulting in increasing cure rates[6].

May 2016

References:

1. Centers for Disease Control and Prevention, "Sexually Transmitted Diseases Treatment Guidelines, 2015," MMWR Reomm Rep 2015; 64(no. RR)
2. Grimes, Jill (Editor) Sexually Transmitted Disease: An Encyclopedia of Diseases, Prevention, Treatment, and Issues, 2014 GREENWOOD, Santa Barbara, Ca. (Vol. 1)
3. Centers for Disease Control and Prevention, "Human Papillomavirus (HPV) Vaccine Safety," http://www.cdc.gov/vaccinesafety/vaccines/hpv-vaccine.html
4. Medline Plus, Hepatitis B Vaccine, http://www.nlm.nih.gov/medlineplus/druginf/meds/a607014.html
5. Center for Disease Control and Prevention, "Hepatitis C FAQs for Health Professionals", http://www.cdc.gov/hepatitis/HCV/HCVfaq.htm Accessed May 2016
6. AASLD/IDSA, "Recommendations for testing, managing, and treating Hepatitis C," http://www.hcvguidelines.org Accessed May 2016

⇨ The above information is reprinted with kind permission from the Medical Institute for Sexual Health. Please visit www.medinstitute.org for further information.

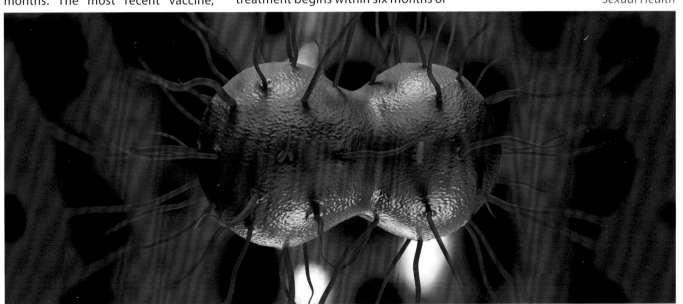

Revealing the truth behind STD and STI myths

An incredible number of myths surround the delicate subject of sexually transmitted infections and diseases (STIs and STDs). According to medical professionals, sexually transmitted infections (STIs) have a high probability of being spread from person to person through sexual contact, but there are cases when other factors can cause the infection.

The term STI is quite broad: some infections are curable and may not cause any symptoms. But if the infection results in altering the typical function of the body, it is then called a disease: STD for 'sexually transmitted disease' or VD for 'venereal disease'.

We want to make sure that our customers are always informed and up-to-date with all factors that can affect their general well being. For this reason, we have put together a list of the most common STD and STI myths. This can help you to tell the difference between what is true and what is not when it comes to this delicate subject.

1. STIs and STDs can only be sexually transmitted

This is perhaps the biggest myth of all. It is the general belief that sex needs to occur and fluids need to be exchanged in order for infections to be passed, because they are called "sexually transmitted".

It is certainly true that you are at a higher risk if you have or have had more than one sexual partner; you also run the risk of becoming infected if you have sex with someone who has had many partners and if you don't use a condom when having sex.

However, for some STIs, no penetration is needed. Germs hide in semen, blood, vaginal secretions and also sometimes in saliva. Some, such as those that cause genital herpes and genital warts, may be spread through skin contact. You can even get hepatitis B by sharing personal items, such as toothbrushes or razors, with someone who has it.

You can also be infected with trichomoniasis through contact with damp objects, such as wet towels, wet clothing or toilet seats, although it is more commonly spread by sexual contact. STIs can also be spread if you share needles when injecting intravenous drugs.

2. You cannot be cured from an STI/STD

Some people believe that you are doomed once you get a sexually transmitted infection or disease. There are different types of sexually transmitted infections, which can be broken down into three basic types: bacterial, viral and parasitic. Bacterial and parasitic infections can be cured. Viral infections can be treated, but not completely cured.

Bacterial STDs include chlamydia, gonorrhoea and syphilis. Viral STDs include HIV, genital herpes, genital warts (HPV) and hepatitis B. Trichomoniasis is caused by a parasite.

3. People get STIs/STDs through same-gender sexual intercourse

There used to be a widespread belief in the 80s and 90s that STIs/STDs only affected homosexuals. However, all three types of infection can occur whether you have heterosexual or homosexual sex.

4. STI/STD symptoms can be easily spotted

Knowing as much as possible about STDs and STIs is one of the best ways to keep yourself sexually healthy. If you are a teenager, it may be helpful to get STI information from an adult, such as a parent, school nurse or teacher.

Sometimes people with STIs do not have any symptoms. If you are not routinely getting tested, you won't know your status. You could unknowingly be passing it onto other partners or the infection could be doing some significant harm to your body. Some of the best tools for prevention and early detection are communicating with partners about their STI status, routine testing and safer sex practices.

5. Self-diagnosis is not dangerous

If you have an STI or STD, you should seek professional medical advice. There are at least 15 fake products being sold online claiming to treat, cure or prevent STDs. While these websites look official and medically informative, you should not trust them. The FDA (The Food and Drug Administration) in the US states that none of these products have been shown to treat any disease and they may have untested ingredients that could cause harm. Effective treatments for sexually transmitted diseases are only available by prescription, from a certified health professional.

The same applies for home treatment: it is never appropriate for STIs. Evaluation by a health professional is needed for any changes or symptoms in the genital area; only an evaluation will suggest an STD or a suspected exposure to an STI.

13 September 2015

⇨ The above information is reprinted with kind permission from the Oxford Online Pharmacy. Please visit www.oxfordonlinepharmacy.co.uk for further information.

© Oxford Online Pharmacy 2017

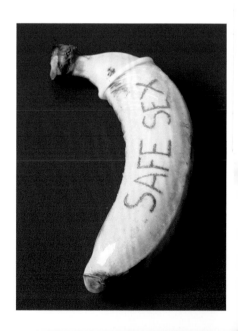

Talking about sex

Children and young people are learning about sex and relationships from soaps, magazines, adverts and their friends. The media is full of confusing messages about sex – it can seem like everyone is doing it all the time.

Talking with their parents helps young people to feel safer and less anxious, allowing them to make up their own minds about the choices they take. It also gives them the confidence to talk to future partners about their relationship, sex and contraception.

Making time to talk shows you are there to support your sons and daughters as they grow up. It does not mean that you are encouraging your children to have sex. All the facts show that if you talk openly about sex, young people delay having sex and are more likely to use contraception. By talking to your children about sex, you can help them to sort out fact from fiction, understand the changes in their bodies, and talk openly about feelings and relationships. They will be grateful to hear about your opinions and beliefs and to have a chance to talk about their own views.

How to talk about sex and relationships

It is important to be open with your children about sex and relationships. Teenagers who talk to their parents about these issues are more likely to be responsible in their relationships and to wait longer to have sex for the first time. They are also more likely to use contraception.

Teenagers learn about sex and relationships in many ways – from their friends, television or the Internet. The different messages they hear can be confusing and that is why it's important for parents to give their teenagers the chance to talk about what they know, or don't know and what choices they have, whatever their own views are.

Young people say they want their parents to talk to them about relationships, responsibilities and values and not just about biology. They may find it hard to talk about or feel embarrassed. Be reassuring,

start the conversation at a time when you are both relaxed and getting on OK, not during an argument or when either of you are feeling annoyed about something. Listen to and talk with them, not at them. If they don't seem ready to talk, don't start nagging or laying down the law. Once you've broken the ice, next time you say something it may be much easier.

All children are different. Adapt how you talk and listen, especially when talking about risky behaviour including sex. Some teenagers prefer reading information whilst others find it easier to talk things through. Most will need more than one conversation. Being open and available when needed is extremely important.

'I said - I'm too young to be a granddad. That got us talking!'

Keep an open mind. Your teenager may be confused about their sexuality and feelings. They may worry that no-one will be interested in them, or that they don't seem to be interested in sex. They may know or think that they are bisexual, lesbian or gay. You may feel shocked, upset or even angry - but they deserve your respect and support whatever your opinion about their sexuality.

Young people often talk about being pressured into early sex and they need help in delaying until they feel it is right for them. Open discussion can help them think things through and give them the confidence to resist these pressures. The majority of young people don't have sex before 16. Those who do are much more likely to regret it and not use contraception. Some parents worry that sex education at school encourages young people to have sex early. There is no evidence that this is the case and there is plenty of evidence that Sex and Relationships Education (SRE) helps young people be more aware of risks and how to make safe choices.

Contraception and safer sex

It is a good idea to start talking about contraception before your children become teenagers if possible. Both

boys and girls have to understand that they must share the responsibility if they decide to have sex, and make sure they are protected from pregnancy and sexually transmitted infections. It's very important for boys and girls to think about what pregnancy means and to know about condoms so they feel confident enough to insist that a condom is used, and comfortable enough to get them from the clinic or the chemist themselves.

"I said - I'm too young to be a granddad. That got us talking!"

Sexual health

Young people need to know how to protect themselves from sexually transmitted infections (STIs) as well as pregnancy. Both boys and girls are vulnerable to HIV and AIDS but they are even more likely to get infections such as chlamydia which can cause infertility if not treated promptly. STIs often have no symptoms so encourage them to get themselves tested and to be responsible for their physical and sexual health.

Parents need to remind young people that only condoms protect against infection. Even if a girl is on the pill it's important to use condoms as well, as the pill will only help prevent pregnancy. By talking about STIs and condoms you and help your teenagers understand the risk and protect themselves.

If there is any possibility that your teenager might have caught an STI, you should encourage him or her to contact your nearest NHS Sexual Health or GUM (Genito-urinary medicine) clinic as soon as possible. Your GP or nurse can give you details. If you would rather keep it private, you can search for the information online.

⇨ The above information is reprinted with kind permission from Family Lives. Please visit www.familylives.org.uk for further information.

© Family Lives 2017

The naked truth about young people's sex lives

Problems with sexual function are often considered an older person's problem, and the assumption still lingers that young people are willing and able to get it on at the drop of a hat. Interest in young people's sexual behaviour tends to focus instead on preventing the spread of sexually transmitted infections, unwanted pregnancies and non-consensual sex.

But a new article drawing on data from the third National Survey of Sexual Attitudes and Lifestyles (Natsal-3), published last week in the *Journal of Adolescent Health*, paints a different picture.

The research, conducted by NatCen, the London School of Hygiene and Tropical Medicine and UCL, revealed that a sizeable minority of young men and women have experienced sexual problems.

More than a third (34%) of sexually active men in this age group had experienced one or more problems with their sexual function, of which over a quarter (27%) said they felt "very" or "fairly" distressed about it. Their most commonly reported problems were reaching climax too quickly, experienced by 13% of men, and lacking interest in sex, experienced by almost 11% of men.

More than a third (34%) of the men who reported reaching climax too quickly were distressed about it, whereas only 13% were distressed by their lack of interest in having sex. Around 8% told us they experienced difficulty getting or maintaining erections, of which 42% were "fairly" or "very" distressed about it. Overall, 6% of men said they had avoided sex in the past year due to a problem with their sexual function.

Compared with men, women in this age group were more likely to have experienced problems with sexual function, and more likely to say they were distressed by it. As many as 44% reported experiencing one or more problems with sexual function, with lack of interest in sex (22%) and difficulty climaxing (21%) the most common problems reported by young women.

Overall, one in three young women who had experienced one or more sexual function problems in the past month said they found this problem distressing. The most distressing problems experienced were among the least common: whilst 8% of young women said they felt anxious during sex, 35% of them reported feeling very or fairly distressed about it. Similarly, 9% of young women reported feeling physical pain as a result of sex, 36% were distressed by it. Around 7% of women reported avoiding sex because of a sexual problem; lack of interest, lack of enjoyment, anxiety and pain were the main reasons given for this.

Despite this, both young men and young women were unlikely to seek help for these problems. Just 36% of men and 42% of women had sought help about their sexual function problems in the past year. Those who did seek help were most likely to turn to family members and friends; just 4% of men and 8% of women with sexual function problems had visited a doctor or other health professional.

This is unsurprising – seeking help for sexual function problems is uncommon even among older adults – but concerning. Studies have also shown that fears about erectile problems among young men contribute to inconsistent condom use and other risky behaviours.

It's also possible that some of these problems, such as anxiety, lack of enjoyment and difficulty in reaching climax, arise due to a lack of positive sex education. A programme of sex and relationships education which emphasises not only the biology of intercourse but also the emotional demands of sexual intimacy and how to make sex pleasurable for everyone involved could go some way to reducing some of these problems.

8 August 2016

⇨ The above information is reprinted with kind permission from NatCen Social Research. Please visit www.natcen.ac.uk for further information.

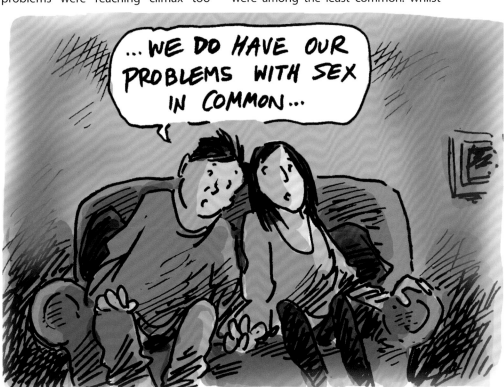

Sexual health services: your rights

When it comes to sexual health services, you have the same rights whether you are over 16 or under 16 and regardless of your sexuality or gender.

This section gives you some information about your rights and the services and standards you can expect both at Brook and elsewhere. It also gives advice on what you can do if you think the services you have received have not been good enough.

Confidentiality

Young people under 16 still have the same rights to confidentiality as anyone else, and you should not be treated any differently.

Doctors and nurses have very strict rules on confidentiality and the law says they have to keep all patient records and information completely private. However, in exceptional circumstances, like when a doctor or health worker thinks you might be in serious danger, they might feel there is a need to pass information on but, even if they do, they must talk to you first before they tell anyone else. This applies to everyone, no matter what age you are.

Government guidance for workers in England means that they are more likely to be more worried about young people under 13 who are having sex, and might think it would be in the young person's best interest to get some extra help from a social worker.

If you are worried about confidentiality you can always call your doctor's surgery without telling them who you are and ask them some questions, like:

⇨ Is the information that I give you kept confidential?

⇨ Do you ever tell anyone else about young people who ask for contraception or advice about sex?

⇨ Would you ever tell anyone else about my visit without telling me first?

Read Brook's privacy and confidentiality policy and guide to NHS sexual health services.

Going to a different doctor

If you need to see a GP, but don't want to go to your usual one, you have the right to consult another doctor.

There could be a number of reasons why you might want to go to a different doctor. You might need to see another doctor if your own one doesn't provide contraception services. You might be feeling embarrassed at the thought of talking to your family doctor about sensitive subjects, like abortion or sexually transmitted infection (STI) testing or, maybe, you just don't like your doctor. Whatever your reason, you have the right to consult another doctor.

You could opt to see another doctor at your GP surgery and you can ask your new doctor not to tell your regular GP that you have been prescribed contraception if you wish. But if you'd prefer to go elsewhere, there are other places you could go. You can go to your nearest Brook service, young person's service, family planning clinic or sexual health clinic and get free and confidential medical advice, contraception and treatment. Read about all the options open to you and what each one is best for.

Contraception

You have the right to speak confidentially with a doctor, nurse or medical professional about contraception as well as to be provided with it. Young people under 16 still have the same rights to confidentiality as anyone else, and you should not be treated any differently.

Government guidance for health workers in England means that they are more likely to be more worried about young people under 13 who are having sex, and might think it would be in the young person's best interest to get some extra help from a social worker.

There are lots of methods of contraception to choose from and different methods suit different people. You can explore our section on contraception but perhaps the best way to find out which methods are most suitable for you is to speak with a doctor or nurse. Find your nearest Brook service.

All contraception is free on the NHS in the UK, so you don't need to pay anything for it.

Medical records

Under the Data Protection Act 1998, you have a legal right to see your medical records.

If you want to see your records ask at your GP surgery and you can arrange a time to go in and read them. Sometimes you might be required to ask in writing. You will usually receive a response to your request within 21 days, although the law states that your hospital, or surgery, has up to 40 days to respond.

You can find more information about seeing your medical records.

Making a complaint

If you're not happy with the care or treatment you've received, or if you've been refused treatment for a condition you have the right to complain and have your complaint investigated.

Most doctors, nurses and health workers want to help you and do all they can to make you feel comfortable when you ask for their advice, but, occasionally things go wrong, or you may feel you have been given bad advice.

You can complain in person or ask someone else you trust, such as a family member or friend, to complain on your behalf. It's best to make your complaint as soon as possible and definitely within six months.

You can complain either to the service that you're unhappy with or you can complain to whoever commissions your local services instead.

You can find more information on how to make a complaint about your healthcare. If you wish to make a complaint about a Brook service you can read our complaints page for further information.

Updated November 2016

⇨ The above information is reprinted with kind permission from Brook. Please visit www.brook.org.uk for further information.

Nearly a quarter of girls in care become teenage mothers, reveals CSJ

⇨ CSJ reveals thousands of cases of children going missing from care each year

⇨ 36 per cent of care leavers are not in education, employment or training (NEET) by age 19

⇨ Create scorecards to name and shame councils failing children in care

⇨ Help care leavers get on in life by funding £2,000 apprenticeship bursaries

Nearly a quarter of girls leaving care become teenage mothers – around three times the national average, according to a new report by a leading think-tank.

The 22 per cent figure means that around 1,000 females from care are becoming teenage mothers every year.

The Centre for Social Justice (CSJ) is concerned about an inter-generational cycle of disadvantage it says is running through England's struggling care system. It has found that at least one in ten care leavers aged 16–21 who are parents have had a child taken into care in the last year.

"When you take children into care you have a unique opportunity to break the cycle of disadvantage – too often this isn't happening," said Alex Burghart, CSJ Policy Director.

"Many parts of the care system are in tatters and we desperately need to rescue it to protect our most vulnerable children."

The think tank says many local authorities are failing in their duty to support young people and build a network of positive relationships around them. It says pregnant teenagers need help to become good parents themselves and this is often lacking.

The figures on teenage parenting represent just one example of a system struggling to look after those in care.

Those leaving the care system are now twice as likely not to be in education, employment or training (NEET) at the age of 19 than the rest of the population.

Symptoms of a system at breaking point are demonstrated in other aspects. Exclusive new figures uncovered by the CSJ reveal thousands of vulnerable children go missing from England's care system on a regular basis.

Local authorities in England reported 252 cases where children have gone missing from care for more than 28 days in the last year. There were 4,452 cases of children missing for more than a day and 707 for more than a week. But only around two thirds of local authorities responded to the freedom of information request so the real number will be much higher.

"If this many children were going missing from their families it would spark national outrage," Mr Burghart added.

"Children in the care system need proper support and protection. We need to learn the lessons of what can happen to children who are not cared for – as we saw in Rotherham."

Teams supporting young people leaving care are often overstretched and unable to build relationships, the report *Finding Their Feet* adds. The average caseload of a personal adviser in some areas is 49 young people.

The CSJ recommends introducing scorecards to highlight which local authorities are failing children and young people from care.

It says there is often a lack of continuity between care workers and young people and recommends overhauling the system and introducing new support networks, based on a similar scheme in the US.

Researchers also call on the Government to end a financial imbalance between care leavers who go to university and those who take on apprenticeships. Currently bursaries of £2,000 are given to those who go to university, but there is no central government equivalent for apprentices. The report says this is an injustice and urges that apprentices also be given a £2,000 bursary.

19 January 2015

⇨ The above information is reprinted with kind permission from The Centre for Social Justice. Please visit www.centreforsocialjustice.org.uk for further information.

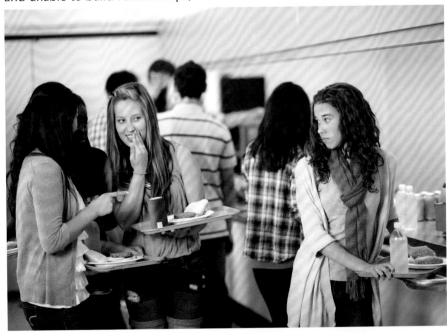

How teenage pregnancy collapsed after birth of social media

Have Facebook and Snapchat helped stop teenagers having sex? New figures show teenage pregnancies plunging to record low since social media explosion.

By John Bingham, Social Affairs Editor

Teenage pregnancy rates have almost halved since the birth of social media as a global phenomenon, official figures show.

The rate of pregnancies among girls under 18 in England and Wales has dropped by 45 per cent since 2007 and now stands at the lowest level since records began almost 50 years ago, according to the Office for National Statistics.

The startling decrease has prompted a host of theories including sex education classes paying off, changing attitudes to young motherhood and the impact of immigration.

But others have speculated that it could be that young people are simply spending less time physically in each other's company because of social media – a phenomenon which went global around 2007, the year after Facebook expanded beyond university campuses.

The drop in teenage pregnancies has been accompanied by evidence of decreases in other traditionally risky behaviours such as drinking and drug taking.

Children's charities and experts have repeatedly warned that the explosion of social media is exposing young people to new dangers from online bullying to 'sexting' and sexual exploitation by strangers.

But the new figures suggest that the change in how teenagers conduct their social lives could also be helping make them safer.

Overall 22,653 girls under 18 got pregnant in England and Wales in 2014 – a drop of almost seven per cent in a single year. Among under-16s it fell by ten per cent in the same period.

The rate of conceptions among under-18s dropped from 41.6 per 1,000 girls in the age-group in 2007 to 22.9 per 1,000 in 2014.

Prof. David Paton, an economist at Nottingham University Business School – who was among the first to suggest a social media effect on pregnancies – said it was striking that a similar pattern is emerging in other countries such as New Zealand.

"It does potentially fit in terms of timing," he said.

"People [appear to be] spending time at home – rather than sitting at bus stops with a bottle of vodka they are doing it remotely with their friends."

He argued that better access to contraception could not explain the fall as it coincides with cuts to sexual health services in many areas amid a period of major austerity.

One other possibility, he said, was that major improvements in schools in areas such as London around the same time might have played a part.

But he added: "Nobody really knows why we've got this sudden change around about 2007 to 2008."

Meanwhile the number of pregnancies among older women rose, continuing a long-term trend towards later motherhood.

Notably, the figures also show that 7.8 per cent of pregnancies involving married women ended in an abortion – the highest level for 12 years.

Yet among unmarried women the abortion rate fell slightly from 31.2 per cent of conceptions to 31 per cent.

Clare Murphy, director of external affairs at the abortion provider British Pregnancy Advisory Service (Bpas) said access to contraception and sex education had "undoubtedly" played a part in the declining teenage pregnancy rate but she agreed with Prof. Paton's suggestion of a social media effect.

"The plummeting level of teenage drinking, for example, may be reducing the likelihood of unprotected sex, and teenagers are also increasingly socialising online, limiting the opportunities for sexual activity," she said.

She added: "As we have seen decreases in conception rates among the under-25s, the largest rise was for women aged 35–39 (a percentage increase of 2.3 per cent).

"Women are increasingly being chivvied about starting their families in their 20s, but the reality is many will wait until their 30s to do so.

"The reasons for this are diverse and will include the time it takes to obtain financial and career security, and not least finding the right person to embark on parenthood with.

"Rather than chastising women, we should support their choices.

"There may be some increased risks with later motherhood, but these need to be kept well in perspective, and women respected as the best judges of when it is best for them to have children."

9 March 2016

⇨ The above information is reprinted with kind permission from *The Telegraph*. Please visit www.telegraph.co.uk for further information.

© *Telegraph Media Group Limited 2017*

The latest statistics on teenage births are missing a vital ingredient: fathers

An article from The Conversation.

THE CONVERSATION

By Maria Lohan, Senior Lecturer in Nursing and Midwifery, Queen's University Belfast and Áine Aventin, Research Fellow in Nursing & Midwifery, Queen's University Belfast

Teenage births are declining across much of the developed world. For example, the latest statistics show teenage births in Northern Ireland, as in the rest of the UK, are experiencing a steady downward trend: from 1,791 in 1999 to 839 in 2014.

However, these figures only tell us about teenage births not teenage pregnancies. We don't know how many teenagers in Northern Ireland have abortions. Restrictions mean most women who wish to terminate a pregnancy travel to other parts of the UK or Europe to do so or obtain 'abortion pills' over the Internet, leaving an incomplete picture of teenage pregnancies.

We do know that the rest of the UK still has one of the highest rates of teenage pregnancy in Europe, despite recent falls. Just under 25,000 women under the age of 18 became pregnant in England and Wales in 2013 and approximately half of these opted for legal abortion. So it is likely that the rate of teenage pregnancy in Northern Ireland is quite a lot higher than the rate of teenage births.

However, the latest figures on births also tell us little about the fathers. Teenage pregnancy is often considered to be a woman's problem, or a problem for women and children – or even society more broadly – but teenage men are rarely part of this picture.

Counting the costs

Of course, not all teenage pregnancies are unintended or unwanted. They can be a welcome and fulfilling aspect of many teenage women's lives. Yet, when we do count the negatives, we only count these in terms of the adverse medical, educational and economic outcomes for teenage mothers and their children.

Also, when we count the costs, it is always in terms of the costs of 'teenage mothers' to the exchequer. For example, we know that every year in England approximately £26 million is paid in benefits to teenage mothers on income support. The Northern Ireland government has pinned the cost to the economy of each teenage mum at £20,000 a year based on income support plus tax revenue foregone with an approximate annual cost to the Exchequer of £25 million.

But most births to teenage women are also births to teenage men. Teenage boys have a vital but neglected role in preventing unintended pregnancy and standing up to the responsibility of dealing with a teenage birth. Research shows children with fathers who are involved in their lives do better in education, are happier (have higher self-esteem and life satisfaction) and have better relationships with childhood friends as well as relationships in adulthood. The children of involved fathers are also less likely to show problem behaviours such as delinquency and other criminal behaviours.

But to help men plan for parenthood in their lives we need to start educating young men at an earlier age. Boys are less likely to receive relationship and sexuality education in schools in general and especially in relation to teenage pregnancy. The lack of resources for teaching boys about teenage pregnancy has prompted the World Health Organisation among others to call for action. And research shows that parents are much less likely to talk to their sons than their daughters about avoiding a teenage pregnancy.

The rates of teenage births are also thought to be much greater for boys and young men who might be most in need of support. Approximately one in four young men in young offenders' institutes are thought to be or about to become fathers.

Part of the solution

It's time to engage teenage men not just as part of the problem of unintended pregnancy in teenagers' lives but as part of the solution. To do this, we should ensure that teenage fathers are always registered as fathers at the birth of their children. We can also provide boys with better relationship and sexuality education, which includes them in the reproductive equation and educates them that as they become sexually active they also become reproductively active too.

Recognising this need, my colleagues and I are studying the effectiveness of a new educational resource entitled "If I were Jack…". This is designed to help young boys aged 14 to 16 years as well as girls imagine the consequences of an unintended pregnancy and to develop the skills to avoid one.

Teenage pregnancy and teenage births are not all about the girl – and forgetting that comes with costs both for our society and for thousands of children. It's time to share the responsibility with young men, from pregnancy to birth to fatherhood.

6 July 2015

Sexually transmitted diseases in older age are an area of neglect

By Prakash Tyagi, Director, GRAVIS

HIV's disconnect with people in older age in terms of programmes, priorities and strategies has increasingly been discussed over recent years. Yet, conversations on sexually transmitted diseases overall remain more neglected.

Despite the vast number and complexity of sexually-transmitted diseases, older age is often considered a stage in the life course when they don't matter.

Syphilis, chlamydia and gonococcal infections have been found to be very common in people over the age of 50, affecting people into their 60s, 70s and beyond.

What contributes to the prevalence of sexually transmitted diseases in older age?

With life expectancy increasing, people are entering their 50s and 60s in much better health and enjoying a longer, more active sexual life. Meanwhile, the risk of infection transmission continues in older age.

Simultaneously, older people's awareness of the wide range of sexually transmitted diseases remains low. There is a link between increasing prevalence and older people's neglect in sexual health education in development programming.

Exacerbating the issue is that many infections, such as syphilis, have a long latency period and may manifest in later stages of life. Further still, sexually transmitted diseases

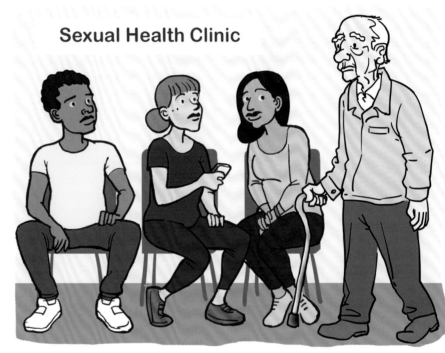

Sexual Health Clinic

can have multiple relapses after a successful cure, reappearing as people age.

As a result, large numbers of older people have to live with the pain and misery of these infections in many communities around the world, particularly in low- and middle-income settings.

The impact on older people

In older age, other medical conditions resulting from and co-occuring with sexually transmitted diseases are common, connected to the particular physiological characteristics and lower immunity related to ageing. This can compound the impact of such infections.

At the same time, older women have to go through more complex challenges of facing stigma from their families and communities.

What can be done?

Education is key to tackling sexually transmitted diseases in older age. It is the missing link in prevention and control programmes.

Yet primary health care services also need to be receptive to the challenge of infection among older people and ensure they are age-friendly in their response.

28 October 2015

⇨ The above information is reprinted with kind permission from HelpAge. Please visit www.helpage.org for further information.

Help Age 2017

Abstinence pledges increase risk of STDs and pregnancy in young women

By Léa Surugue

Young women who break an abstinence pledge may be more at risk of unwanted pregnancies and sexually transmitted diseases (STDs) than peers who have never taken such a pledge in the first place, scientists claim. In the United States, about 12% of adolescent girls vow not to have sex before marriage, but up to 88% of them end up breaking this promise.

In a study published in the *Journal of Marriage and Family*, scientists have analysed the health data of more than 20,000 American teenagers to assess the impact that taking a virginity pledge has on female sexual health. In particular, they wanted to determine whether 'pledgers' were less likely to become pregnant outside marriage or to test positive for a common STD – the human papillomavirus (HPV).

In the US, sexual education is often a source of controversy. The CDC recommends in-school programmes focusing on the prevention of STDs and pregnancy, including educating on condom use. The problem is that this initiative is not always well accepted. In fact, only about half of high schools and one-fifth of middle schools provide sexual health education that meets CDC criteria, with abstinence often being the only other alternative presented to teenagers.

By identifying a high risk of pregnancies outside marriage and significant rates of HPV in pledge-breakers, the latest research provides new critical evidence that abstinence-only policies are not effective to promote healthy sexual behaviours in adolescents.

HPV screening and pregnancies

Scientists looked at data from a nationally representative, longitudinal study of adolescents. These included information collected between 1994 and 1995 when 20,745 students in grades seven to 12 – between 13 and 18 years old – answered questions regarding their health, romantic relationships and whether they had taken abstinence pledges.

Between 2001 and 2002, 15,197 of them were re-interviewed. The researchers specifically focused on female participants, looking at their HPV screening results and whether they had become pregnant at any time outside marriage. They then compared the results of women who had never taken an abstinence pledge and those who did, but ended up breaking it.

Overall, HPV rates did not differ significantly, with about a quarter of girls testing positive in each group. However, when the researchers focused on young women who had had two or more sex partners, pledge-breakers tested positive for HPV in higher proportions. Additionally, 30% of pledge-breakers – compared to 18% of non-pledgers – became pregnant outside marriage, in the six years after they began having sex.

Dangers of abstinence only policies

According to the authors, these findings suggest young girls who have broken an abstinence pledge may engage in riskier sexual behaviours than girls who never vowed abstinence.

They may be less prepared and less aware of how to deal with the risks of sexual activity, because abstinence policies often go hand-in-hand with a rejection of condoms and other contraceptives. Since a majority of pledgers break their promise to stay virgins until marriage, this can have important, unintended health consequences.

"If adolescents either are provided inaccurate information about condom use or contraception or are socialised to be hostile to these practices, they could be in a bind when they break pledges, as almost all of them do," the scientists conclude.

4 May 2016

⇨ The above information is reprinted with kind permission from IBTimes. Please visit www.ibtimes.co.uk for further information.

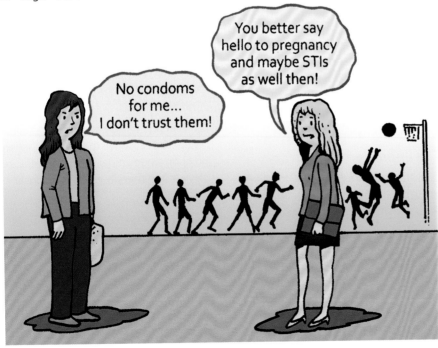

Have young people stopped fearing sexually transmitted infections?

***An article from* The Conversation.**

THE CONVERSATION

By Rosie Webster, Research Associate in Digital Health and Sexual Health, UCL

The good news is that rates of teenage pregnancies are at record lows. In 2014 in England and Wales they were at the lowest rate since 1946, with only 15.6 pregnancies per 1,000 women younger than 20.

Unfortunately, rates of sexually transmitted infections (STIs) are still very high. There were 440,000 diagnoses in the UK in 2014, and the under-25s are one of the most high risk groups. STIs have a high financial cost for testing and treatment: diagnoses of chlamydia alone cost the NHS £620 million in 2011.

Condoms provide effective protection against STIs but many people choose not to use them – around [15% of under-25s](http://www.thelancet.com/pdfs/journals/lancet/PIIS0140-6736(1362035-8.pdf) reported having unprotected sex with two or more partners in the last year. So why don't young people use condoms? The most commonly given reason is the impact on sexual pleasure [and intimacy](http://www.jahonline.org/article/S1054-139X(0300137-X/abstract). Pleasure is of course a very important part of sex, so anything that is perceived to interfere with it is bound to be viewed negatively.

Mixed evidence

Some also argue that young people don't use condoms because they aren't scared of contracting STIs anymore. Today, the majority of common STIs, including chlamydia and gonorrhoea, can be cured quickly with antibiotics, while HIV can be managed and those who contract it can expect to live 20 years longer than was the case in 2000.

While this idea makes sense, the evidence supporting it is mixed. Research has shown people's beliefs about the seriousness of non-HIV STIs are not related to their behaviour, suggesting that it doesn't make any difference whether people think

STIs are serious or not: they're still likely to put themselves at risk. This is despite the fact that, if left untreated, they can cause complications such as infertility.

Fear of HIV, on the other hand, may well influence behaviour. The problem is that many people may not feel at risk of catching it, particularly non-black-African heterosexual people, who are statistically at lower risk of HIV. One study showed heterosexual people who were at high risk of STIs and HIV underestimated that risk and many didn't use condoms. This suggests that young people's decision to use a condom or not may depend on whether they think they are at risk of an STI rather than how severe they think the consequences are.

We should also be aware that the decision to wear a condom isn't always made by one person. Their partners may also be involved, and expectations about their reaction (or a lack of discussion altogether) may influence the choice. Getting caught in the "heat of the moment" is a commonly cited barrier to condom use and experiments have shown that sexual arousal in men reduces their ability to make decisions.

Sex-positive approach needed

So what can we do to change this situation? Previous educational programmes have often focused on the "dangers" of unprotected sex. But evidence suggests that scaring people, in particular those who feel unable to change their behaviour, can just cause them to become defensive.

The fact that perceived loss of sexual pleasure appears to be the fundamental reason most people don't use condoms highlights how important it is to address the positive aspects of sex, rather than solely focusing on the negative consequences. Finding a way to enhance sexual pleasure with

condoms, or at least change beliefs about pleasure, is important. This could be as simple as improving actual sensation with condoms, from recommending thinner designs to revolutionary new materials such as graphene. Alternatively, it could involve persuading people that safe sex can be good sex.

This sex-positive approach attempts to target an important driver of behaviour: motivation. We are primarily driven by our wants and needs in any particular moment. Therefore, we need to make people want to use condoms, rather than making them feel that they should. To do this, we should focus on outcomes that are important to people – things that we know they want.

For example, when targeting smoking, focusing on appearance-related consequences may be more effective than focusing on health-related consequences, for people who value being attractive. Interventions to increase condom use should therefore focus on more immediate goals that young people care about, such as enjoying good sex or gaining social approval.

We certainly haven't cracked the problem of getting people to use condoms yet. However, focusing on goals that are important to young people create an exciting new area for future investigation.

29 July 2015

⇨ The above information is reprinted with kind permission from *The Conversation*. Please visit www.theconversation.com for further information.

Should the NHS pay for HIV-prevention drug?

By John Humphrys

A high court judge has ruled that the National Health Service has responsibility for deciding whether or not to supply a drug called PrEP that helps prevent the transmission of HIV, the virus that causes AIDS.

The decision has been hailed as a victory by gay campaigners. But others argue that the NHS should be spending its scarce resources on what they regard as much more urgent and deserving treatments. Who is right?

Despite the impression created by some newspaper headlines, the judge, Mr Justice Green, did not order the NHS freely to prescribe pre-exposure prophylaxis (PrEP) to all gay men who want it so that they can practise unsafe sex. He was adjudicating a much narrower legal point, which followed from the decision of the Coalition Government to hive off responsibility for public health from the NHS to local authorities.

The NHS, which initially said it was prepared to consider prescribing PrEP, had changed its mind because, it said, it did not have the legal right to do so and it was the responsibility of local council. This was challenged in court by the National Aids Trust and the NAT won.

NHS England said it would appeal against the ruling, but it also raised the temperature by putting out a statement that was seen as highly controversial. It said that it had to ration its spending and could not confirm funding for other highly expensive treatments. They include treatment for cystic fibrosis in children, low sodium levels in the blood of chemotherapy patients and brain implants for children with hearing problems. Deborah Gold, of the NAT, said it was "deeply unhelpful" of NHS England "to be pitting PrEP against other treatments".

However, if NHS England loses its appeal, then making a decision between providing one treatment rather than another is exactly what the NHS will have to do, simply by virtue of the fact that the NHS does not have the money to provide for free every treatment that medical science comes up with. Rationing is a fact of life in the NHS and what the judge has decided is that the NHS must include PrEP when it is calculating what it will and what it won't prescribe.

Those who support the prescribing of PrEP say it's pretty much an open-and-shut case. The drug has been shown to reduce the risk of transmission of HIV by around 86%. The number of new cases of HIV in Britain has been rising each year and PrEP's success rate offers the best chance available to reverse the trend radically. They also argue that it is highly cost-effective. The treatment costs around £5,000 a year per patient. It's reckoned that on average the treatment would need to be prescribed only for about two years to each patient, making a total cost of around £10,000 a patient. This compares with the average lifetime cost of treating someone with HIV of £360,000. Furthermore, the cost of the drug, provided by the pharmaceutical company Gilead, is likely to fall dramatically when the patent runs out in 2018.

Nonetheless, the cost to the NHS over the next couple of years of prescribing PrEP would be around £20 million a year and the benefits of not having to fork out for lifetime HIV treatment would accrue only over a much longer period. So, given the cash shortage in the NHS in the immediate future, opponents argue it should concentrate its limited resources on more deserving treatments than PrEP.

At the heart of their case is the distinction they draw between illnesses that afflict people through no cause of their own and those that are the consequences of the lifestyle choices they make. In this context HIV is very much seen as an illness that is the consequence of choice: the choice of whether or not to practise safe sex. Using a condom has been shown to be the safest way to avoid the transmission of HIV and condoms are freely available on the NHS. So why, the argument goes, should the NHS spend £20 million a year on a drug simply so that those who don't like using a condom can have sex without running the risk of catching or transmitting HIV? Surely it is obvious, they say, that that £20 million should be spent instead on, say, the budget for a drug that treats the faulty gene in some children with cystic fibrosis (annual cost of £182,625 per treatment).

But critics of this line of argument say that the NHS cannot start deciding whether or not to treat somebody on the basis of whether it thinks their

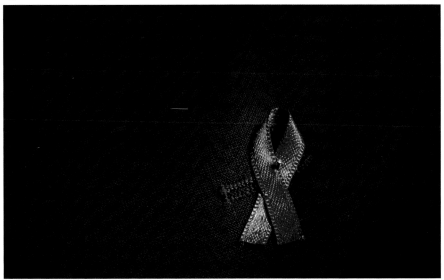

need for treatment is the result of lifestyle choices they make. If that were the criterion, they argue, then smokers should be denied treatment when they develop lung cancer, and the obese should be turned away when they contract diabetes. The NHS has never operated on this basis, they say, and should not start to do so now.

Yet people still need to be encouraged to take responsibility for their own health and opponents of the free prescription of PrEP argue that it would actually discourage responsibility. Their case is that promiscuous gay men, the category most likely to make use of PrEP, would be liable to regard PrEP as a "magic pill" protecting them from HIV. This would encourage them to abandon safe sex and throw away their condoms. But the result of this would be a rise in the incidence of other sexually transmitted diseases (putting further pressure on the NHS). Furthermore, given the fact that PrEP does not give 100 per cent guarantee of protection from HIV, its prescription, if followed by the abandonment of safe sex, could well lead to an increase in HIV, or at least to no appreciable decrease. This in turn would upturn the claim that prescribing PreP would ultimately save the NHS money.

One proposal being suggested is the American approach. PrEP should be available to anyone who wants it but they should pay for the pills themselves rather than require the NHS to pick up the tab. To many people, however, this would be yet another case of undermining the founding principle of the NHS – that treatment should be available free at the point of use.

Mr Justice Green has lobbied the decision of whether PrEP should be available free of charge back into the NHS court. What decision do you think the NHS should take?

4 August 2016

⇨ The above information is reprinted with kind permission from YouGov. Please visit www.yougov. co.uk for further information.

Call to extend cervical cancer vaccine to boys

Boys should be given a cervical cancer vaccine only given to girls to protect them against infectious diseases.

The BMA annual consultants conference in London today agreed the UK HPV (human papillomavirus) Gardasil vaccination programme should be extended to boys to provide protection against various cancers.

Consultants said this could also improve population-wide immunity.

Girls are offered the vaccine at the age of 12 or 13 to protect them against cervical cancer. The Gardasil vaccine protects them against genital warts, which are caused by some types of HPV.

International evidence

London GUM consultant Eleanor Draeger told the conference that Australia, Canada and the US had extended their Gardasil vaccination programme to boys after an Australian audit showed it reduced the incidence of genital warts in girls exponentially.

She said doing so in the UK would provide greater protection through herd immunity.

Dr Draeger said: "It is fair to say that there is some [existing] herd immunity for straight men because if the girls were vaccinated then straight men will be protected.

"There is, however, no herd immunity for straight men who have sex with older women, who are not protected because they weren't vaccinated because they've missed the vaccination programme, or for men who have sex with men."

She added it would also help reduce rates of particular types of cancer.

Outrageous risk

Dr Draeger said: "The incidence of anal carcinoma in men who have sex with men is as high as the incidence of cervical cancer in women before the advent of the cervical screening programme. It is outrageous that they are not being protected.

"When a survey was done of consultant GUM physicians 61 per cent [of those who had children] said that they were planning to pay privately to have their boy children vaccinated.

"Australia, Canada and the US have already extended their vaccination programme to boys and I believe that we should as well."

Fife public health medicine consultant Charles Saunders added: "If we want rid of HPV as a serious problem, vaccinate boys too."

BMA consultants committee joint deputy chair Sara Hedderwick said vaccination was cheap but also easy to cut as a cost-saving measure.

She said the vaccine should be extended to boys to ensure protection for all.

30 June 2016

⇨ The above information is reprinted with kind permission from the BMA. Please visit www.bma. uk for further information.

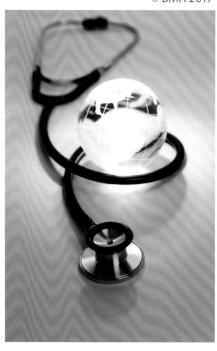

Council cuts hitting women's contraceptive services, data shows

Advisory Group on Contraception warns that reducing sexual health services could lead to a rise in unintended pregnancies and abortions.

By Denis Campbell

Clinics offering women contraception are closing or reducing their opening hours in the wake of heavy Whitehall cuts to local councils' public health budgets, new research has revealed.

One and a half million women of reproductive age live in parts of England where councils have restricted contraception services or are considering doing so, according to data obtained under freedom of information by the Advisory Group on Contraception.

The findings have prompted warnings from sexual health experts that paring back such services could lead to an increase in unintended pregnancies and abortions. One in four councils have already reduced their contraception service or may do so, the new findings show.

"Councils are between a rock and a hard place when faced with cuts to public health budgets, but it's a false economy to restrict women's access to contraception," said Natika Halil, the chief executive of the Family Planning Association, which is a member of the AGC.

She cited research showing that every pound spent on contraception saved £11 in averted health costs, for example from women going on to have a baby or a termination.

"Making it harder for women to choose the right contraception for them will mean more unplanned pregnancies and more abortions," she said.

Four sites offering contraception services have closed or will close during 2016–17 in Dorset and several clinics have stopped operating in Wandsworth in south London.

Responses from 140 of England's 152 councils to the freedom of information requests showed that a lunchtime school drop-in service in south Gloucestershire has been ended, a sexual health worker in Wokingham in Berkshire lost their job when a condom distribution service was brought in-house by the council and a young people's service in Bexley, south London, ceased being a standalone service but is now being provided in a local GP's surgery.

Dr Anne Connolly, a GP in Bradford who sits on the AGC, said: "It's hugely concerning to see that, in many parts of the country, contraceptive services are being cut, meaning that women can't access the most reliable types of contraception. Without close scrutiny, I'm worried this trend will only continue and that women will bear the consequences."

Among the 140 councils which responded, 20 (14%) confirmed that at least one site had shut in 2015–16 or would do so this year, while another 18 (13%) said that clinics could be closed this year. The AGC is made up of health charities such as the FPA, doctors, the Local Government Association and the Faculty of Sexual and Reproductive Healthcare, which represents specialists.

Councils in England have been obliged by law since the Coalition Government's NHS shake-up in 2013 to provide open access to sexual health services, including for contraception.

NHS England commissions some contraceptive services under its contract with GPs. The AGC also found that fewer councils now have contracts with local family doctors to provide the long-acting forms of contraception that women are now often encouraged to use.

However, councils have had to reduce the public health services they offer since the Treasury cut £200 million from their budgets for this year and it intends to take another £600 million by 2020–21, just under 10% of the planned total.

Simon Stevens, the chief executive of NHS England, has warned several times that cuts to public health will inevitably lead to higher long-term costs for the NHS. Last year, he said he was "crystal clear that any further cuts in public health and social care would impose extra costs on the NHS over and above the minimum funding requirement [the £8 billion extra by 2020–21 that then chancellor George Osborne promised last year to give the NHS]".

The Department of Health said councils were best at deciding what public health services they provided for their residents.

"Local areas are best placed to decide how to provide the sexual health services their communities need. Good progress is being made; for example, teenage pregnancy is down 30% in England since 2011, the lowest for 40 years," a spokesman said.

"Over the next five years, we will invest more than £16 billion in local government public health services, in addition to what the NHS will continue to spend on vaccinations, screening and other preventative interventions."

* This article was amended on 13 December 2016. An earlier version said a sexual health clinic operating at Leighton hospital in Crewe, Cheshire, was shut down last year. It has been relocated to a nearby site.

12 December 2016

⇨ The above information is reprinted with kind permission from *The Guardian*. Please visit www.theguardian.com for further information.

Drunk or flirty rape victims often 'to blame,' says survey

Official government figures show teenagers and older people are more likely to say sex attack victims who had been drinking, flirting or taking drugs were at least partly responsible.

By David Barrett

More than a quarter of the public believe drunk victims of rape or sexual assault are at least partly responsible for what has happened to them, official figures show.

The Office for National Statistics (ONS) published research which also showed more than a third of interviewees insisted sex attack victims bore partial responsibility if they had been "flirting heavily" beforehand.

Teenagers and the 55 to 59 age group were less likely to be sympathetic to sex attack victims who had been drinking or flirting than people in their 20s, 30s and 40s, the poll showed.

Among 16- to 19-year-olds 34 per cent said a victim's drunkenness made them "completely", "mostly" or "a little" responsible, along with nearly 46 per cent who said the same about a victim who had been flirting with their attacker.

In comparison, only 24.5 per cent of people aged 20–24 agreed on the drunkenness question, and 39.7 per cent on flirting.

Among a slightly older age group, the 25- to 34-year-olds, the figures were 22.4 per cent and 29.5 per cent respectively.

Women's groups said the findings were of "great concern" because they showed younger people were more likely to "make excuses for perpetrators".

The findings will trigger further debate about the role of consent in rape cases and other sexual assault prosecutions, just two weeks after the Director of Public Prosecutions set out new guidelines on the subject.

Alison Saunders, who heads the Crown Prosecution Service, said defendants accused of rape should always be asked to prove how they knew their alleged victim was consenting.

The issue of consent has been highlighted by the rape conviction of Ched Evans, the former Sheffield United striker, in April 2012 for raping a 19-year-old waitress, who was judged to be too drunk to consent to sex.

The release of Evans last year triggered a row over his bid to return to professional football and its possible effect on young people as a role model, despite the 25-year-old Welshman maintaining his innocence.

It was the first time the ONS research, from the Crime Survey for England and Wales, had asked in such detail about the public's attitudes towards victims of sexual assault.

The poll also found 31 per cent of people thought victims were at least partly to blame if they had been taking drugs.

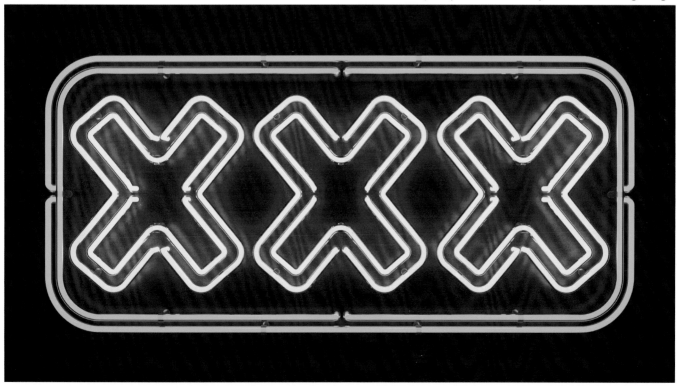

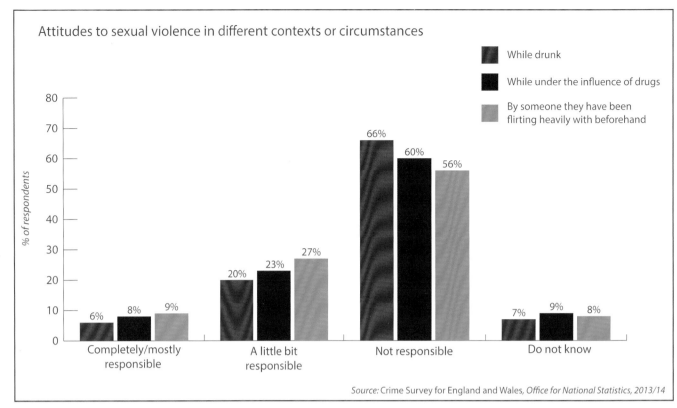

Attitudes to sexual violence in different contexts or circumstances

Legend:
- While drunk
- While under the influence of drugs
- By someone they have been flirting heavily with beforehand

% of respondents

Completely/mostly responsible: 6%, 8%, 9%
A little bit responsible: 20%, 23%, 27%
Not responsible: 66%, 60%, 56%
Do not know: 7%, 9%, 8%

Source: Crime Survey for England and Wales, *Office for National Statistics, 2013/14*

Again, teenagers were more likely to apportion blame to the victim, at almost 45 per cent, compared with just over 25 per cent of those aged 25 to 34.

Sarah Green, director of the End Violence Against Women Coalition, said: "We already know that a significant minority of the population are inclined to blame women for being raped, but what should be a cause of great concern in these figures is the fact that younger people are significantly more likely to blame women and girls for rape.

"Research by the Children's Commissioner on young people's understanding of consent showed that most were aware of the law on rape, but that when presented with different real-life rape scenarios most tended to deny it was rape and to blame the women and make excuses for perpetrators.

"Young people today are bombarded with confusing and conflicting messages about men and women and sexuality in popular culture – women are constantly portrayed as sex objects and it is implied that it is 'natural' for men to pursue women to the point of coercion."

A spokeswoman for the Women Against Rape campaign group said: "Too often, judges and others in authority make derogatory remarks about victims. This has an impact on how others view victims.

"We believe that every age group needs to stop blaming women for rape and putting responsibility directly onto the rapist."

12 February 2015

⇨ The above information is reprinted with kind permission from *The Telegraph.* Please visit www.telegraph.co.uk for further information.

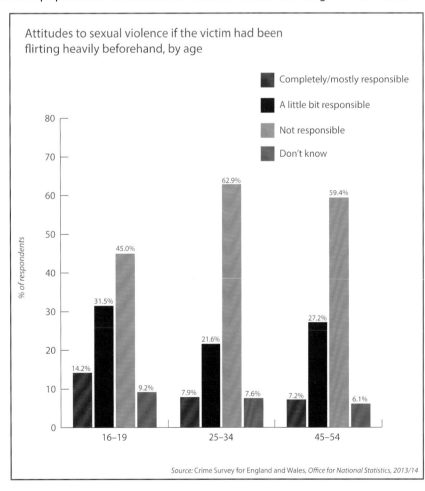

Attitudes to sexual violence if the victim had been flirting heavily beforehand, by age

Legend:
- Completely/mostly responsible
- A little bit responsible
- Not responsible
- Don't know

% of respondents

16–19: 14.2%, 31.5%, 45.0%, 9.2%
25–34: 7.9%, 21.6%, 62.9%, 7.6%
45–54: 7.2%, 27.2%, 59.4%, 6.1%

Source: Crime Survey for England and Wales, *Office for National Statistics, 2013/14*

40% of teenage girls pressured into having sex

Physical violence and abuse also a factor in 20% of relationships, new research finds.

Research published today reveals that more than four in ten teenage schoolgirls in England* have experienced sexual coercion. Most were pressured to have sex or other sexual activity, but some cases included rape.

Controlling online behaviour by partners, through constant checking of their social network activity, sending threatening messages or telling them who they could be 'friends' with was closely associated with young people experiencing violence or abuse from their partner offline.

Pornography influencing teen attitudes to sex and relationships

The researchers found that a high proportion of teenage boys regularly viewed pornography and one in five harboured extremely negative attitudes towards women.

Almost four in ten (39%) boys in England aged 14–17 admitted they regularly watched pornography and around one-fifth (18%) strongly agreed with statements such as:

⇨ "It is sometimes acceptable for a man to hit a woman if she has been unfaithful." Boy, aged 14–17.

⇨ "Women lead men on sexually and then complain about the attention they get." Boy, aged 14–17.

Pressure to send sexual images

England had the highest rate for children exchanging sexual images and messages with a partner among the countries surveyed.

More than four in ten (44%) girls and just under a third (32%) of boys in England had sent them to their boyfriend or girlfriend. Just over 40% of girls who sent them said they had been shared by a partner with others.

Just under half of girls and boys in England had received them. Around a quarter (27%) of girls sent messages and images because they felt pressurised by a partner to do so.

Young people who reported violence and abuse in their relationships were at least twice as likely to have sent a sexual image or text compared to those who had not.

Girls who took part in the survey said:

⇨ "I've had relationships where I wouldn't be able to go out with my friends because they'd get angry with me. I have been raped and other things like that." Kate, aged 15.

⇨ "He breathed down my neck 24/7, it was horrible." Amy, aged 15.

Sex education urgently needs updating

We are calling on the Government to take action to ensure teenagers get a clearer message about healthy relationships.

Claire Lilley, head of child safety online said:

"The levels of victimisation revealed by this research shows action is urgently needed by the Government to make updated sex and relationship education a statutory right for every child and young person. There needs to be a greater focus in schools on topics such as sexual exploitation and violence against girls and young women, as part of a balanced curriculum.

"The high rates of sexual coercion discovered need to be addressed through education and awareness-raising that challenges attitudes and helps change behaviour. We need to nurture children to have positive relationships based on mutual respect.

The highest rates of sexual coercion were reported by teenage girls in England. Around one in five (22%) also said they had suffered physical violence or intimidation from boyfriends, including slapping, punching, strangling and being beaten with an object. In interviews with 100 of the children, many said the pressure to have sex was so great it almost became "normal" and in some cases rape was not recognised.

The research in England was undertaken between 2013–2015 by a team of researchers from the Universities of Bristol and Central Lancashire led by NSPCC Senior Research Fellow, Dr Christine Barter.

The study was also carried out in Norway, Italy, Bulgaria and Cyprus, as well as England. It is one of the biggest of its kind ever undertaken in Europe, involving a school-based survey of 4,500 children and 100 interviews with young people.

Lead author Dr Barter, who is based at Bristol's School for Policy Studies, said:

"Our research findings show that across Europe violence and abuse, both offline and online, in young people's relationships constitutes a major problem, yet in most countries it remains unrecognised leaving young people with little support or appropriate services."

Nicky Stanley, Professor of Social Work at the University of Central Lancashire and co-author, commented:

"Teenage girls reported serious distress and harm following abusive behaviour from boyfriends. Education and campaigns need to challenge stereotypical behaviour and attitudes in boys, and the law in this area should be clearly communicated to young people, their parents and teachers."

The research was funded by the Daphne III European Commission.

*1,001 young people were surveyed in England

⇨ The above information is reprinted with kind permission from the NSPCC. Please visit www.nspcc.org.uk for further information,

© NSPCC 2017

Half of Indian girls don't know about menstruation until they get their first period

Though 28 May is observed as Menstrual Hygiene Day, studies find that periods are still a taboo for most women across the world.

By Bismah Malik

In India, nearly half the girls don't know about menstruation until they get their period for the first time, a recent research has showed. The study, published in the *British Medical Journal* (BMJ) in March 2016, involved 100,000 adolescent girls, among which only half the girls knew about menstruation before they got their periods.

According to the study, the use of sanitary napkins was more prevalent among girls in urban areas than among those in rural areas. Inadequate disposal of used pads was widespread. The study also found that menstruating girls in India faced many religious restrictions.

Despite women spending a considerable part of their lives menstruating, it turns out that most of them still consider periods as taboo. According to UNICEF, menstruation is still not talked about. It can be seen as dirty or impure and the silence around it can lead to a lack of knowledge, which can generate damaging misconceptions,UNICEF said in an official statement.

Although 28 May is observed every year as Menstrual Hygiene Day, and is aimed to raise awareness among men and women, a research done by Carla Pascoe from the University of Melbourne said that menstrual blood is still a cause of embarrassment to many women, ABC.net reported.

Pascoe studied the changing attitudes of women towards menstruation over the past century by interviewing women across various age groups, and found one thing constant – period shame. She, however, said that over the years, the taboo has become subtle and complex.

She also said that although hygiene seems to be no longer an issue among women, as most of them are now familiar and equipped to manage "that part of the month," women however still feel the need to hide their blood stains, and used tampons.

Pascoe's research identified that the single most important factor that determines the reason behind period shame is that money can still be made by promising women effective ways to hide period blood. "If you analyse the advertisements from sanitary product companies, most of them are 'buy our product because we can offer you a more effective way to conceal menstruation'," Pascoe was quoted by ABC.net as saying.

The study also found that women could go to any length to hide their period blood.

"Women told me if they go to someone's house and there is no bin in the bathroom, they would bundle up a pad or tampon into toilet paper and stick it in their bag and take it home – these are grown women," she said.

The study's findings raise an alarm, especially when various international agencies have been urging women to adopt a more confident attitude towards menstruation.

28 May 2016

⇨ The above information is reprinted with kind permission from *IBTimes*. Please visit www.ibtimes.co.uk for further information.

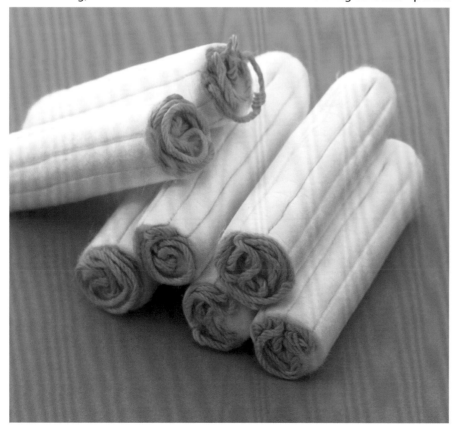

School is now young people's main source for sex information

School is the main source of information about sex and relationships for more young people than ever before, academics have found. However, a majority of young people feel they are not getting all the information they need.

The findings have come from the third National Survey of Sexual Attitudes and Lifestyles and the research has been conducted by University College London (UCL), the London School of Hygiene and Tropical Medicine, and NatCen Social Research.

The academics compared the data from nearly 4,000 young men and women aged 16 to 24, which was taken between 2010 and 2012, with that from previous surveys in 1990-91 and 1999–2001.

The analysis shows that for both men and women, school is now the most commonly reported main source of information about sexual matters, having risen from 28 per cent in 1990 to 40 per cent in 2012.

Parents, on the other hand, were the main source for just seven per cent of the young men and 14.5 per cent of the young women. Meanwhile, health professionals were the main source for one per cent and three per cent respectively. Other sources included:

⇨ First sexual partners: 12 per cent of men and five per cent of women.

⇨ Friends: 24 per cent of men and women.

⇨ Siblings: Two per cent of men and women.

⇨ Media sources: Seven per cent of men and eight per cent of women.

⇨ Pornography: Three per cent of men and 0.2 per cent of women.

Researchers found that both men and women who learned about sexual matters mainly from school first experienced sexual intercourse at a later age and were less likely to report unsafe sex or getting sexually transmitted infections (STIs).

The findings also show a gap between the information young people wanted and what they received in school – with young men in particular missing out.

Young people specifically said they wanted more information about "sexual feelings, emotions and relationships", as well as STIs, and for women, contraception.

When asked for their preferred source of additional information, young people most commonly said school (46 per cent of men and 49 per cent of women), followed by parents (37 and 46 per cent), and health professionals (22 and 27 per cent).

One of the study's authors, Wendy Macdowall, a lecturer at the London School of Hygiene and Tropical Medicine, said: "Our results suggest we need a broader framing of sex education in schools that addresses the needs of both young men and women, with a move away from the traditional female-focused 'periods, pills and pregnancy' approach.

"Our research from Natsal is timely with the current debate on sex and relationships education (SRE) in schools, but it's also important to remember that introducing statutory SRE

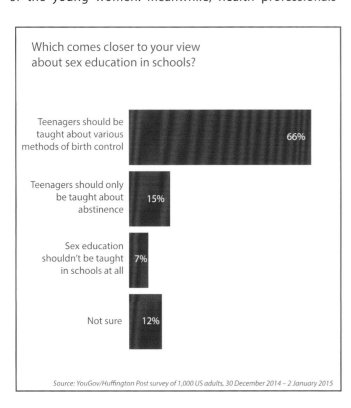

Which comes closer to your view about sex education in schools?

- Teenagers should be taught about various methods of birth control: 66%
- Teenagers should only be taught about abstinence: 15%
- Sex education shouldn't be taught in schools at all: 7%
- Not sure: 12%

Source: YouGov/Huffington Post survey of 1,000 US adults, 30 December 2014 – 2 January 2015

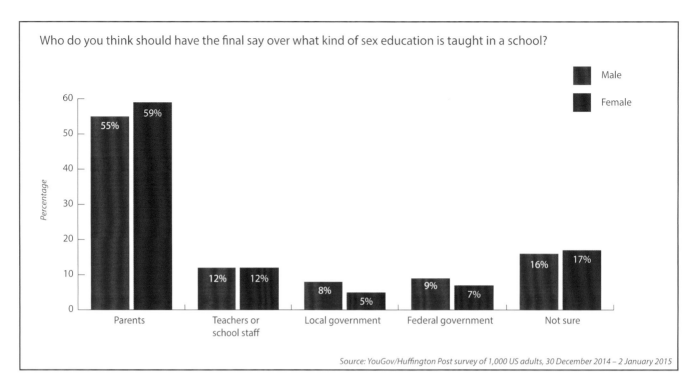

Who do you think should have the final say over what kind of sex education is taught in a school?

- Male
- Female

Percentage

	Parents	Teachers or school staff	Local government	Federal government	Not sure
Male	55%	12%	8%	9%	16%
Female	59%	12%	5%	7%	17%

Source: YouGov/Huffington Post survey of 1,000 US adults, 30 December 2014 – 2 January 2015

in schools won't solve everything. The factors influencing poor sexual health are multiple and complex and so too must be the solutions to them."

Fellow author, Dr Clare Tanton, senior research associate at UCL, added: "The terrain young people have to navigate as they are growing up has changed considerably over the past 20 years and it will inevitably continue to do so. This means that while we need a more structured approach towards SRE, we must also be able to adapt to these changing needs.

"The fact that many young people told us they wanted to get more information from a parent shows that parents also have an important role to play. There needs to be a combined approach which also supports parents to help them take an active role in teaching their children about sex and wider relationship issues."

Commenting on the findings, Jane Lees, chair of the Sex Education Forum, said: "This study powerfully illustrates the difference it can make when young people have reliable sources of information about sex and relationships. Good quality SRE needs to be universal in schools and meet the needs of boys as well as girls.

"We urge all political parties to make a manifesto commitment to statutory SRE. Parents need support too so that they can play their role in talking to their children. Boys in particular are missing out on conversations about growing up at home.

"If legislation is changed and SRE becomes compulsory in all primary and secondary schools there will be fresh scope for partnership between school and home so every child is guaranteed age-appropriate and reliable information about relationships, their bodies and sex."

12 March 2015

⇨ The above information is reprinted with kind permission from SecEd. Please visit www.sec-ed.co.uk for further information.

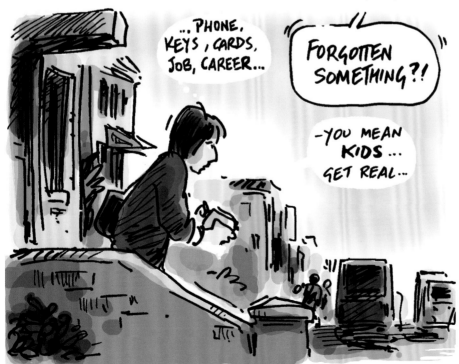

Children should be shown pornography and sex education should be abolished, says Dame Jenni Murray

"Why not teach them how to analyse it?"

By Amy Packham

Dame Jenni Murray has called for changes to the education system, including "abolishing" sex education and introducing "gender lessons".

The Radio 4 presenter, 66, said school children should watch pornography and "analyse it" – just like they would do with a book in an English lesson.

"I would abolish sex education," she said during the Cheltenham Literature Festival, according to the Daily Mail. "I would put the 'what goes where and how and how things are made' and all of that into biology because that is science and no parent is going to say: 'Oh, I don't want my child getting involved in biology or science.'

"What we would then have is a compulsory subject called gender education, so it doesn't have the word sex in it so nobody can complain or be upset."

Murray said allowing children to watch pornography would get them thinking about what they are actually watching.

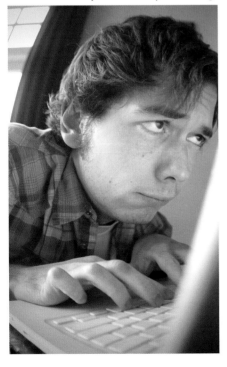

She added: "Why not show them pornography and teach them how to analyse it?

"So then at least those girls know and all those boys know that normal women do not shave, normal women do not make all that noise those women make, they are making all that noise because they need a soundtrack on the film."

The 66-year-old also said pornography is easily accessible – something she believes parents are unaware of.

She said parents should talk to their children about it and not assume they're not watching it.

When asked to comment on Jenni Murray's speech, Lisa Hallgarten, co-ordinator of the Sex Education Forum, told The Huffington Post UK: "The Sex Education Forum welcomes the growing chorus of people from across the political and professional spectrum, including Jenni Murray, calling for more and better sex education in schools.

"We want comprehensive sex and relationships education in every school in the country. Young people say they want to learn about healthy relationships, gender issues, safety and emotional well-being alongside the biological aspects of puberty, sex, sexual health and reproduction."

An NSPCC spokesman said: "Jenni Murray is right that children's access to internet porn is having a damaging impact on their understanding of sex and relationships. But to suggest we scrap sex education lessons and show them porn in school is highly irresponsible and parents will be rightly appalled at her comments.

"The solution is twofold. Firstly children need to be prevented from viewing adult porn.

"Secondly, we all need to understand how viewing porn can have a damaging impact on young people's lives, and the NSPCC wants porn to be discussed as part of age-appropriate sex and relationships education – in fact we want this to be a compulsory part of the national curriculum rather than leaving it to the discretion of individual schools."

Mumsnet CEO, Justine Roberts, told HuffPost UK: "What parents on Mumsnet have consistently and strongly called for is compulsory and comprehensive sex and relationships education to address things like porn, consent and sexting head-on starting in primary school in an age-appropriate way.

"Watching porn at school is probably a large step too far for many parents (let alone non-specialist teachers), but the ability to engage critically with the adult material they see all around them is an increasingly important skill for teenagers."

The National Curriculum in the UK for sex education is compulsory from age 11 onwards.

"It involves teaching children about reproduction, sexuality and sexual health. It doesn't promote early sexual activity or any particular sexual orientation," the Government website states.

12 October 2016

⇨ The above information is reprinted with kind permission from The Huffington Post UK. Please visit www.huffingtonpost.co.uk for further information.

Young people say that sex and relationships education in schools is negative and out of touch

By Roger Pebody

A review of 55 separate studies of sex and relationships education (SRE) in schools shows that young people have many criticisms of its narrow approach and its delivery by poorly trained, embarrassed teachers. Classes focus on avoiding unwanted pregnancy and sexually transmitted infections, but give little attention to the needs of lesbian, gay, bisexual and transgender (LGBT) pupils.

"SRE should be 'sex-positive' and delivered by experts who maintain clear boundaries with students," the researchers write in *BMJ Open*. "Schools should acknowledge that sex is a special subject with unique challenges, as well as the fact and range of young people's sexual activity, otherwise young people will continue to disengage from SRE."

Background

In England, local-authority run state schools must teach anatomy, puberty, the biological aspects of sexual reproduction, sexually transmitted infections (STIs) and HIV/AIDS. Schools are not obliged to teach any other aspects of sex and relationships education. Moreover, academies, free schools and private schools are not obliged to provide any SRE at all.

Requirements differ in Wales and Northern Ireland. In Scotland, schools are not obliged to provide any SRE at all.

The quality of SRE is thought to vary widely. Quantitative studies conducted with young people indicate that SRE starts too late, is too biological, doesn't cover all relevant issues, has a negative tone and is poorly delivered.

The Terrence Higgins Trust, NAT (National AIDS Trust) and Sex Education Forum are campaigning for SRE to be made compulsory in all schools and for it to address the needs of LGBT pupils.

In order to understand the issue in more depth, researchers from the University of Bristol identified previously published qualitative studies of young people's

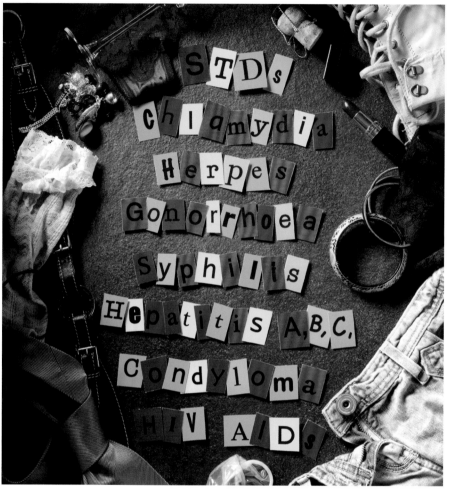

views about the SRE they had received. The researchers used techniques of meta-ethnography and thematic analysis to bring together and synthesise the findings from the original studies.

Most studies were of school-based SRE delivered to secondary school pupils by teachers. Just under half the studies were from the United Kingdom, with most of the others from English-speaking countries in North America or Australasia. In most of the studies, young people took part in focus groups.

Sex as a distinctive issue

An over-arching theme was that schools have taken insufficient notice of the distinctive nature of sex as a topic. Sex is a potent subject that can arouse strong emotions and reactions, but schools seem to deny that there is anything exceptional about the topic. They attempt to teach

SRE in the same way as other scientific subjects.

Students reported embarrassment and discomfort, particularly in mixed-sex classes. While young men are expected to be sexually knowledgeable, they were afraid of revealing themselves as sexually inexperienced by asking a question, as this pupil explained:

"Some people are too scared to say things so they cover that up by being noisy and disrupt the class."

Young women often took SRE classes seriously but in mixed classes, male pupils sometimes discouraged their participation by verbally harassing them. Teachers often failed to confront young men about this kind of behaviour.

Young people wanted to receive SRE in a safe and confidential environment that would allow them to participate without inhibition. Those teachers who were able to maintain control of the class and protect students from ridicule helped pupils engage with the subject. Setting ground rules for discussion, behaviour and confidentiality was seen to be helpful.

Young people criticised SRE for being overly biological, judging the approach to be basic, repetitive, narrow and irrelevant. A Canadian pupil said:

"Everything we got in our class had a really clinical feel, it's just like information but it's not related to yourself."

SRE was also seen to try to contain sexuality within an implicit moral framework. Young people noted a focus on unwanted pregnancy, STIs and the casting of young men as sexual predators. Young people's sexuality was seen as a 'problem' to be managed.

"All they ever do is talk about the dangers of sex and that, and nothing about the pleasure."

A common theme in studies was that homosexuality was barely mentioned, making lesbian, gay, bisexual and transgendered students invisible. Young people wanted homosexuality to be discussed within SRE, to help normalise same-sex relationships, address homophobia and support young LGBT people.

Out of touch with pupils' lives

Schools appear to struggle to accept that some young people are sexually active. This leads to SRE content that is out of touch with many student's lives. Many young people reported that SRE was provided too late, when they were already having sex.

With SRE narrowly focused on heterosexual intercourse, young people said that it didn't acknowledge the full range of sexual activities they engaged in – many of which would actually be counted as 'safer sex'. A pupil in Northern Ireland said:

"So you just were taught about sexual intercourse causing pregnancy, but you were never taught about masturbation; you were never taught about oral sex and all the different, other types of sexual practices…"

Young people wanted classes to talk more about what sex involves and how to have sex. Many young men were

anxious about being able to 'perform' and particularly wanted this information. As it wasn't provided, many turned to pornography instead.

Many wanted to know how to make sex pleasurable but this wasn't discussed. Female pleasure was particularly absent from SRE, reproducing stereotypes of women as passive and lacking in desire. Young women also wanted to talk about emotions and relationships.

"They don't really go into the whole relationships thing partly because I don't think – they don't want us to have relationships."

"They didn't talk about the emotional part of having sex. They didn't really talk about how sex will affect you as a person and how it affects your emotions."

Since schools have difficulty accepting young people's sexuality, SRE failed to discuss some issues that were relevant to sexually active young people – the health services they can use, their options available if pregnancy occurred, and the pros and cons of different contraceptive methods.

Who should provide SRE?

Teachers were commonly reported to be embarrassed and awkward when delivering SRE. Students reported that teachers seemed unable to discuss sex frankly and responded unsatisfactorily to questions. Teachers were thought to be poorly trained on the issue.

"If your teacher who's a grown up can't talk about it, how are you [supposed to]? That gives you the impression that, oh I'm not really supposed to talk about it."

While it's often thought that teachers are well-placed to deliver SRE because they know their students, it was this familiarity that many students found inappropriate. It disrupted existing relationships and breached boundaries – it was embarrassing to discuss sexual matters with teachers they would interact with again in the future.

The power imbalance between pupils and teachers also inhibited discussion.

When SRE had been delivered by peer educators, students reported more egalitarian and mutually respectful relationships. They felt a sense of affinity with the peer educators, which encouraged them to believe the information they provided. Young people

appreciated the techniques they used to create a safe environment and their use of discussion-based approaches.

Many young people liked the idea of sexual health professionals delivering SRE. They were perceived to be less judgemental and better informed than teachers. As with peer educators, their lack of experience in maintaining classroom discipline could sometimes be a problem. But both peer educators and sexual health professionals had the advantage of not having an ongoing relationship with pupils.

"You want someone who's not from the school or someone who actually does it as a job and knows what they're talking about and you know can be professional about what they are telling you."

Conclusion

"Young people's aspirations for SRE appear to align with a 'sex-positive' approach that aims for young people to enjoy their sexuality in a way that is safe, consensual and healthy," the researchers say.

They say it is also important to identify the right educators to deliver SRE. While this review of studies highlights considerable problems with using teachers, the researchers acknowledge practical problems with having SRE delivered by non-teachers. Outside experts are expensive, while peer educators have to be regularly trained as existing cohorts get older. Teachers are seen as a more sustainable option.

The researchers suggest a compromise – specialist SRE teachers who only teach SRE and whom students would not encounter in other contexts. This could address pupils' need for clear boundaries and for skilled providers.

Reference

Pound P et al. What do young people think about their school-based sex and relationship education? A qualitative synthesis of young people's views and experiences. BMJ Open 6:e011329, 2016. (Full text freely available online).

4 October 2016

⇨ The above information is reprinted with kind permission from NAM Publications, 2016. Please visit www.aidsmap.com for further information.

Sex education is letting British teenagers down

An article from **The Conversation.**

By Max Biddulph, Associate Professor, Faculty of Social Sciences, University of Nottingham.

The UK Government has been heavily criticised after rejecting a recommendation for statutory inclusive sex and relationship education in schools. This comes after Office for National Statistics figures recently revealed that in the 12 months to March last year, 30% of female rape victims were aged under 16, a quarter were 14 or younger, and nearly 10% were nine or younger.

Despite MPs' calls for sex and relationship education to be mandatory in all schools, its "non-statutory" status – coupled with the fact that many schools are emerging via the process of "academy-isation" – means that currently schools embrace sex education with varying degrees of enthusiasm. Consequently, it is almost impossible for the subject to be taught at a consistent level across the UK.

The case for making sex education compulsory seems to be more compelling than ever. And in the wake of high-profile child abuse cases in Rotherham and Rochdale, calls have been for a greater discussion of issues of consent for all young people, and young women in particular.

Issues highlighted in recent research undertaken by the Sex Education Forum into young people's experience of sexual education shows there needs to be more focus on the safety around the exchanges of digital images between pupils – with discussions needed on the impact 'sexting' has on young people.

It is also important to evolve the understanding of 'relationships' to include same-sex relations – with young gay and bisexual men particularly poorly served by school sex education classes, in part due to low levels of knowledge around safer behaviour and HIV.

Facts of life

Prior to the Government's decision on sex and relationship education, four different chairs of House of Commons Committees – education, health, home affairs and business – wrote to education secretary Nicky Morgan, saying personal, social, health and economic education, which includes sex education, was a "crucial part of preparing young people for life".

"It can provide them with the knowledge and confidence to make decisions which affect their health, well-being and relationships, now and in the future," said the joint letter.

In her reply to Neil Carmichael – chairman of the education select committee – Nicky Morgan defended the lack of change. She implied schools are either not ready, or do not have the expertise to deliver such classes – with Ofsted finding that 40% of personal, social, health and economic education teaching in schools is less than good.

But strangely, governments have never held back on introducing educational initiatives in the past. In fact, the mandatory nature of the changes often provides a powerful imperative for implementation. A good example is the curriculum reforms in the 1990s, which foregrounded literacy and numeracy.

Beyond the banana

In a lot of ways, sex education is still stuck in the past – when it sought to "regulate the moral and sexual behaviour of citizens in accordance with reoccurring social agendas". This includes encouraging a heterosexually envisaged future, stable family life, the prevention of "promiscuity", and stemming sexually transmissible infections and "unplanned" pregnancies. Unfortunately, this isn't really representative of the age we live in now.

Influenced by the ideas of the eugenics movement, early sex education also sought to encourage "good breeding" to "strengthen the nationhood".

As the situation stands, it seems as though Nicky Morgan is caught in a trap between her own personally supportive position and the potential challenges which might emerge from certain faith groups – who have a vested interest in protecting a more conservative concept of "sexuality". So if sex education was to become compulsory it could create confrontation and a conflict of values.

We need to look deeper at our society and the moral meanings that are attached to sexuality, sexual behaviour and sex and relationship education. Because it is society at large and young people specifically who continue to pay the price for inadequate, patchy sex education. Instead of being seen as "contaminating knowledge", sex education should be seen as a facilitator of individual growth and empowerment. Sexuality, arguably, is a central experience of being human after all.

23 March 2016

⇨ The above information is reprinted with kind permission from *The Conversation*. Please visit www.theconversation.com for further information.

© 2010–2016, The Conversation Trust (UK)

Heads or tails?

What young people are telling us about SRE.

SRE is slowly improving

The survey included the question 'Please give a rating for your school SRE as a whole'

⇨ 22% of respondents rated their school SRE overall as either "bad" or "very bad".

⇨ Just 10% rated it as "very good".

However, male respondents were more likely than female respondents to rate their school SRE as "good" (29%) or "very good" (15%). Respondents identifying as trans, non-binary or other were least likely to rate their SRE as "good" or "very good"; 84% of these respondents rated their school SRE as "OK", "bad" or "very bad".

"In the past years in school I have never had SRE" (Male, 13 years old)

"Sex was still regarded as a taboo subject and the teachers seemed uncomfortable talking about it. The whole concept was approached purely biologically with no regards to relationships at all and was pushed into a few lessons at the end of term alongside drugs education." (Male, 15 years old)

The Sex Education Forum has carried out surveys with young people in 2008, 2011, 2013 and 2015. In each case we have included a standard question asking young people to rate the quality of their school SRE overall. In each case the survey involved at least 800 self-selected young people. While comparisons must be treated with caution (because the cohort varies when using a self-selected sample) there is a trend towards less young people rating their SRE as 'bad' or 'very bad' and more young people rating their SRE as 'good' or 'very good'.

Inequality in SRE provision puts children at risk

The survey included four questions which asked specifically about topics covered at primary school and focused on information that helps a child recognise the difference between behaviour that is and is not sexually abusive and how to get help.

⇨ Just over 70% of respondents ticked that they had learnt correct names for genitalia (e.g. penis and vagina) and that these parts of the body "are private to you".

⇨ 16% had not learnt the correct names for genitalia at primary school.

Looking at respondents who had most recently left primary school this decreased to 10% for respondents aged 11, 12 and 13 years old, suggesting that correct names for genitalia are more likely to be taught in primary schools now than in the past, but leaving 1 in ten respondents who have left primary school in the last three years without basic vocabulary for describing sexual parts of the body.

Learning in primary school about the difference between safe and unwanted touch was much lower than learning about correct names for genitalia.

⇨ Overall, only 40% of respondents had learnt "about the difference between safe and unwanted touching"

⇨ 34% had learnt "how to get help if you experience unwanted

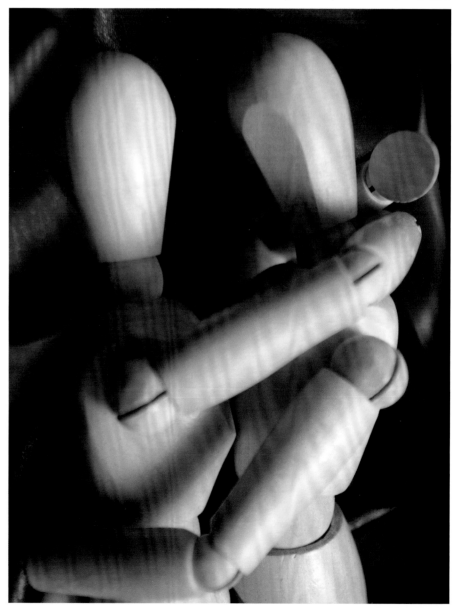

touching/sexual abuse", 50% had not learnt about this and a further 18% were either "unsure" or could not remember.

Amongst the youngest respondents (aged 11, 12 and 13 years old) the levels of learning on these issues were a little higher but within this age group 31% had not learnt "how to get help if you experience unwanted touching / sexual abuse".

Young people were more likely to have learnt about the difference between safe and unwanted touch from discussions at home (45%) than in school (40%), but home cannot be relied upon as 38% of respondents said they had not learnt about the difference between safe and unwanted touch from discussions at home.

Learning (or not) about safe and respectful relationships

The survey included a further set of questions which asked about specific topics covered at school, either primary or secondary, and whether or not these topics were adequately covered. Questions covered both healthy and abusive relationships, sexual consent and pleasure.

⇨ 53% of respondents had not learnt about "how to recognise when someone is being groomed for sexual exploitation" (increased to 86% for young people aged 20–25 and reduced to 33% for young people aged 11–13)

⇨ 46% had not learnt about "how to tell when a relationship is healthy"

⇨ 44% had not learnt about "how to tell when a relationship is abusive"

⇨ 50% had not discussed scenarios that helped you to consider real-life situations to do with sexual consent

⇨ 34% had not learnt about sexual consent

⇨ 48% did not learn all that they needed to about sexual consent

⇨ 43% had not learnt about "the responsibility for getting consent as well as the choice to give consent"

A Sex Education Forum survey of over 800 young people carried out in 2013 and published in January 2014 found that 30% of young people had not learnt about sexual consent in school compared with 34% in this survey.

Questions were included about sexual pleasure. This is an aspect of education about sex and relationships that young people have said is often completely neglected.

⇨ 60% had not learnt about sexual pleasure

⇨ 65% did not learn all they needed to about sexual pleasure

These findings paint a picture in which a young person's chances of learning about safe and respectful relationships in school are about 50/50. Learning about sexual pleasure is even less likely.

Learning about female genital mutilation (FGM)

Young people were also asked if they had learnt about female genital mutilation (FGM) at either primary or secondary school.

⇨ Overall, just 24% of young people said they had learnt about FGM

⇨ 7.6% did not understand the question

⇨ Amongst the youngest respondents (aged 11, 12 and 13) 40% had learnt about FGM and 14% did not understand the question.

An open text comment box was included after the question on FGM and comments included:

"We should have learnt about this"
(Male, 15 years old)

"I'm in year 10 and I don't even know what that is"

(Female, 14 years old)

Discussions with parents and carers at home

Young people were little more likely to discuss safe and respectful relationships at home than they were at school:

⇨ 46% of respondents had not discussed with a parent or carer "how to tell when a relationship is healthy"

⇨ 48% had not discussed "sexual consent" with a parent or carer

⇨ 49% had not discussed with a parent or carer "how to tell when a relationship is abusive"

⇨ 66% had not discussed sexual pleasure

2016

⇨ The above information is reprinted with kind permission from the National Children's Bureau. Please visit www.sexeducationforum. org.uk for further information.

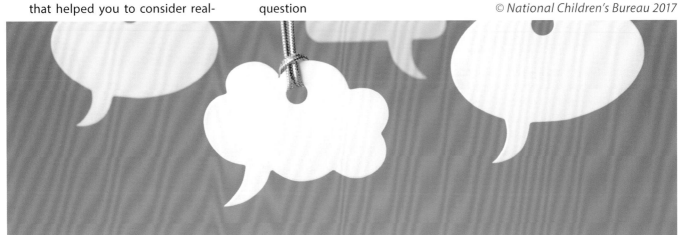

All children need to learn about sexual consent – it's their right

Half the female victims of sexual assault are under 16. Rape victims are most likely to be aged 15 to 19. Schools need to teach young people about healthy relationships.

By Laura Bates

The Government has announced that it will not make sex and relationships education (SRE) compulsory in all schools, flying in the face of advice from experts and pleas from teachers , pupils and parents alike. The decision comes in spite of support for compulsory SRE from key House of Commons committees – the chairs of the education, health, home affairs and business committees all wrote to education secretary Nicky Morgan pressing for the subject to be made statutory in primary and secondary schools, saying it was a "crucial part of preparing young people for life".

But perhaps what is most significant of all is that the decision to reject compulsory SRE came in the very same week that new figures were released by the Office for National Statistics (ONS) revealing that, in the 12 months to March last year, 30% of female rape victims were aged under 16, a quarter were 14 or younger and nearly 10% were nine years old or younger.

Campaigners have long argued that compulsory SRE could be a vital preventative tool to help tackle the wider problem of the 85,000 women raped and 400,000 sexually assaulted in England and Wales every year. But, coupled with the news that such a large proportion of rape victims are children themselves, the case for good-quality sex education becomes even more urgent. To reject an opportunity to give all our children simple, age-appropriate information about their rights over their own bodies, the meaning of consent and their responsibilities towards others, in the very same week that we learn that rape victims of both sexes are most likely to be aged between 15 and 19, is devastating.

In addition to the data on rape, the figures also reveal that half of female victims of other sexual offences, such as assaults, grooming and sexual exploitation, were girls under 16. This completely shatters the argument that we shouldn't teach young people SRE because we don't want to "give them ideas" about adult issues to which they are not yet exposed.

In fact, last year it was revealed that more than 5,500 alleged sex crimes in UK schools had been reported to the police over the previous three years, including nearly 4,000 physical sexual assaults and more than 600 rapes.

Failing to educate young people about sexual consent and healthy relationships means that those who experience such crimes at a young age are often left bewildered, afraid, ashamed and unsure of where or how to report what has happened.

For example, analysis of the Crime Survey for England and Wales, which was published alongside the statistics, showed that respondents in younger age groups were much more likely to think it was acceptable, at least some of the time, to hit or slap their partner if they had an affair. And results from the most recent British Social Attitudes Survey reveal that young people are also significantly more likely than the general population to believe a rape victim is fully or partially responsible for their own assault if they have been drinking, or flirting with their attacker before the incident.

It is so rare, when dealing with issues as ingrained and insidious as sexual violence, to be able to point to concrete solutions that could make a real difference. And yet, in compulsory, good-quality SRE, we have a robust, tangible solution that experts, survivors, young people and educators alike agree could have a major impact.

To reject it is quite simply to fail young people.

It fails the one in 20 children in the UK who already experience sexual abuse, and the one in three children sexually abused by an adult, who do not tell anyone about it.

It fails the 43% of young people who say they are never taught about relationships at school at all, and the 40% who described their SRE provision as either "poor" or "very poor".

It fails LGBTQIA young people who deserve to be informed and included, not alienated and excluded.

It fails the one in three girls who experience unwanted sexual touching (a form of sexual assault) in UK schools.

It fails the 30% of female rape victims aged under 16, who might never be told that what happened to them wasn't acceptable, and that they have the right to report it.

But, most of all, it fails every child who has a human right to learn about sexual consent and their rights to their own body. What lesson could possibly be more important than that?

19 February 2016

⇨ The above information is reprinted with kind permission from *The Guardian*. Please visit www.theguardian.com for further information.

Key facts

- Over the 1990s, NatSal saw an increase in the number of opposite-sex partners people reported, and more people reporting same-sex experience. Over the last decade, NatSal have only seen further increases for women, so the gender gap is narrowing. (page 4)

- According to a NatSal survey, more than 60% of people reported having sex recently and over 60% of people said they were satisfied with their sex life. People in poorer health were less likely to have had sex recently, and less likely to say that they were satisfied. (page 5)

- According to a NatSal survey, around one in 100 people aged 16–44 had chlamydia, although this varied by age, peaking at almost one in 20 women aged 18–19 and one in thirty men aged 20–24. (page 5)

- More than one million sexually transmitted infections (STIs) are acquired every day worldwide. (page 9)

- Each year, there are an estimated 357 million new infections with one of four STIs: chlamydia, gonorrhoea, syphilis and trichomoniasis. (page 9)

- More than 500 million people are estimated to have genital infection with herpes simplex virus (HSV). (page 9)

- More than 290 million women have a human papillomavirus (HPV) infection. (page 9)

- The majority of STIs have no symptoms or only mild symptoms that may not be recognised as an STI. (page 9)

- STIs such as HSV type 2 and syphilis can increase the risk of HIV acquisition. (page 9)

- More than a third (34%) of sexually active men have experienced one or more problems with their sexual function, of which over a quarter (27%) said they felt "very" or "fairly" distressed about it. (page 16)

- As many as 44% [of women] reported experiencing one or more problems with sexual function, with lack of interest in sex (22%) and difficulty climaxing (21%) the most common problems reported by young women. (page 16)

- 8% of young women said they felt anxious during sex and 35% of them reported feeling very or fairly distressed about it. (page 19)

- Nearly a quarter of girls leaving care become teenage mothers – around three times the national average, according to a new report by a leading think-tank. (page 18)

- Teenage births are declining across much of the developed world. For example, the latest statistics show teenage births in Northern Ireland, as in the rest of the UK, are experiencing a steady downward trend: from 1,791 in 1999 to 839 in 2014. (page 20)

- In 2014 in England and Wales [teen pregnancy rates] were at the lowest rate since 1946, with only 15.6 pregnancies per 1,000 women younger than 20. (page 23)

- A poll has showed that teenagers and the 55 to 59 age group were less likely to be sympathetic to sex attack victims who had been drinking or flirting than people in their 20s, 30s and 40s. (page 27)

- Among 16- to 19-year-olds 34 per cent said a victim's drunkenness made them "completely", "mostly" or "a little" responsible, along with nearly 46 per cent who said the same about a victim who had been flirting with their attacker. (page 27)

- Almost four in ten (39%) boys in England aged 14–17 admitted they regularly watched pornography and around one-fifth (18%) strongly agreed with statements such as:

  - "It is sometimes acceptable for a man to hit a woman if she has been unfaithful." Boy, aged 14–17.

  - "Women lead men on sexually and then complain about the attention they get." Boy, aged 14–17. (page 29)

- More than four in ten (44%) girls and just under a third (32%) of boys in England [have sent sexual images] to their boyfriend or girlfriend. Just over 40% of girls who sent them said they had been shared by a partner with others. (page 29)

- The highest rates of sexual coercion were reported by teenage girls in England. Around one in five (22%) also said they had suffered physical violence or intimidation from boyfriends, including slapping, punching, strangling and being beaten with an object. (page 29)

- In India, nearly half the girls don't know about menstruation until they get their period for the first time, a recent research has showed. (page 30)

- Parents are the main source of information about sexual matters for just seven per cent of the young men and 14.5 per cent of the young women. (page 31)

- 22% of respondents [to a recent survey] rated their school SRE overall as either "bad" or "very bad". Just 10% rated it as "very good". (page 37)

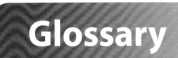

Cervical cancer

Cancer that develops in a woman's cervix (the entrance to the womb from the vagina). In its early stages it often has no symptoms. Symptoms can include unusual vaginal bleeding which can occur after sex, in between periods or after menopause. The NHS offers a national screening programme; a 'smear test' for all women over 24 years old.

Condoms

A thin rubber (latex) sleeve worn on the penis. When used correctly, condoms are the only form of contraception that protect against pregnancy AND STIs. They are 98% effective – this means that two out of 100 women using male condoms as contraception will become pregnant in one year. You can get free condoms from sexual health clinics and some GP surgeries.

Contraception

Anything which prevents conception, or pregnancy, from taking place. 'Barrier methods', such as condoms, work by stopping sperm from reaching an egg during intercourse and are also effective in preventing sexually transmitted infections (STI's). Hormonal methods such as the contraceptive pill change the way a woman's body works to prevent an egg from being fertilised. Emergency contraception, commonly known as the 'morning-after pill', is used after unprotected sex to prevent a fertilised egg from becoming implanted in the womb.

Contraceptive implant

A small flexible tube about the size of a matchstick inserted by a doctor under the skin of a female's upper arm. The device releases hormones to prevent the ovaries from releasing eggs. Lasts for three years, but can be removed before then if the woman decided she wants to get pregnant.

Contraceptive injections

An injection offers eight to 12 weeks protection against pregnancy, but not from sexually transmitted diseases (approx. 99% effective). It works by thickening the mucus in the cervix, which stops sperm reaching the egg, and it also thins the lining of the womb so that an egg can't implant itself there.

Diaphragms

A rubber dome-shaped device worn inside the vagina which creates a seal against the walls of the vagina. It must be inserted before sexual intercourse and must remain in places for up to six to eight hours afterwards. The diaphragm does not provide protection from sexually transmitted diseases.

Emergency contraception

Sometimes referred to as the 'morning-after pill', this is a form of emergency contraception which can be taken by girls within 72 hours after unprotected sex (although preferably within the first 24 hours). It should not be used as a regular method of contraceptive. It is available across the counter at chemists or from your local GP, family planning clinic or sexual health clinic.

Femidom

Female condom: used by the female partner to provide a physical barrier that prevents sperm from reaching the egg. Can help prevent pregnancy and reduce the risk of STIs.

HPV vaccination

An injection for girls which can help prevent cervical cancer and genital warts. The vaccine protects against the two strains of HPV (human papilloma virus) responsible for more than 70% of cervical cancers in the UK. It is most effective a few years before a girl becomes sexually active. A national vaccination programme launched in 2008 to vaccinate 12- and 13-year-old girls.

Safe sex

Being safe with sex means caring for both your own health, and the health of your partner. Being safe protects you from getting or passing on STIs and from unplanned pregnancy.

Sexual health

Taking care of your sexual health means more than being free from sexually transmissible infections (STIs) or not having to face an unplanned pregnancy. It also means taking responsibility for your body, your health, your partner's health and your decisions about sex.

Sexually transmitted disease

A disease or infection that is transmitted through the exchange of bodily fluids such as semen or genital fluids.

The pill

A tablet taken each day, at the same time, by girls to prevent pregnancy. The pill contains hormones that prevent the ovaries from releasing an egg. It only protects against pregnancy and not STIs.

Assignments

Brainstorming

⇨ What is included in the term 'sexual health'?

⇨ What kind of sexual health services are available in your local area?

Research

⇨ Choose one of the contraception methods from the article on pages six, seven and eight. Research it further and create a leaflet listing how it works, as well as its pros and cons.

⇨ Conduct an anonymous questionnaire to find out what your peers think about sex education in your school. You should aim to find out whether they think it is useful, up-to-date and appropriate. You should also aim to find out whether there is anything your peers think should be covered at school that, currently, is not. When you have gathered your results, write a report that summarises your findings. Include graphs and tables.

Design

⇨ Choose one of the articles from this book and create an illustration that highlights the key themes of the piece.

⇨ Design an app for young people that gives details of the most common STIs. See page 11 for help.

⇨ Design a website aged at over 50s explaining the risks of STDs and how to prevent them.

⇨ Create a leaflet that could be displayed in a local GP's office explaining peoples' rights to sexual health services in the UK. Use the article on page 17 if you need help.

⇨ Create an informative leaflet about the different kinds of sexually transmitted infections (STIs), including how they are passed on, symptoms and how to treat them.

Oral

⇨ Read the article *How teenage pregnancy collapsed after the birth of social media* on page 19, then in small groups discuss the possible theories and links between social media and teenage conception rates.

List the theories and write some bullet points under each argument, then share them with the rest of your class.

⇨ Read the article *Should the NHS pay for HIV-prevention drug?* and stage a class debate to argue this question.

⇨ Create a PowerPoint presentation that will explain the issue of consent to a class of fourteen-year-olds. Remember the age of your audience and target your material appropriately.

⇨ As a class, discuss whether you think pornography should be shown as part of sex education lessons.

⇨ Chlamydia is the most common sexually transmitted infection amongst young people. Create an informative presentation on the signs and symptoms of chlamydia, the risks associated with it and how somebody can request a free test kit.

⇨ At what age should sex education be taught? How young is too young? Debate this as a group.

Reading/writing

⇨ Write a one-paragrph definition of the term 'sexual health' and then compare it with a classmate's.

⇨ Write a blog post from the point of view of a fourteen year old giving advice to their parent/caregiver about how they should approach talking about sex. For example, the fourteen-year-old might want the parent to 'just be honest and open' or might say 'don't nag', etc.

⇨ Write a letter to the BMA explaining why you think the HPV vaccine should be extended to boys. Do some research about the history behind the HPV vaccine and use this to inform your letter.

⇨ Write an open letter to your local MP explaining why it is important for women's contraceptive services to remain funded. See the article on page 26 for help.

⇨ What is the definition of rape? Look at sex and the law in the UK. What are the possible consequences of sex or physical closeness without consent? Consider not just the legal impact, but the health and emotional effects too. Write a summary of your findings.

⇨ Sexual health is not just all about STIs; it should also include a respectful understanding of sex and the mental and emotional aspects involved. Make a list of all the things a person should consider before having sexual intercourse.

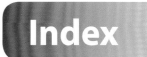

Acknowledgements

The publisher is grateful for permission to reproduce the material in this book. While every care has been taken to trace and acknowledge copyright, the publisher tenders its apology for any accidental infringement or where copyright has proved untraceable. The publisher would be pleased to come to a suitable arrangement in any such case with the rightful owner.

Images

All images courtesy of iStock.

Icons

Icons on page 4 & page 5 (top) were made by Freepik from www.flaticon.com. Icons on page 5 (bottom) were made by Popcorn Arts from www.flaticon.com.

Illustrations

Don Hatcher: pages 3 & 22. Simon Kneebone: pages 16 & 32. Angelo Madrid: pages 1 & 21.

Additional acknowledgements

Editorial on behalf of Independence Educational Publishers by Cara Acred.

With thanks to the Independence team: Mary Chapman, Sandra Dennis, Jackie Staines and Jan Sunderland.

Cara Acred

Cambridge, September 2017